Science of Spices and Culinary Herbs

Latest Laboratory, Pre-clinical, and Clinical Studies

(Volume 3)

Edited by

Atta-ur-Rahman, *FRS*

*Kings College, University of Cambridge, Cambridge,
UK*

M. Iqbal Choudhary & Sammer Yousuf

*H.E.J. Research Institute of Chemistry,
International Center for Chemical and Biological Sciences,
University of Karachi, Karachi,
Pakistan*

Science of Spices & Culinary Herbs

Volume # 3

Editors: Prof. Atta-ur-Rahman, Prof. M. Iqbal Choudhary & Dr. Sammer Yousuf

ISSN (Online): 2590-0781

ISSN (Print): 2590-0773

ISBN (Online): 978-981-14-6836-0

ISBN (Print): 978-981-14-6834-6

ISBN (Paperback): 978-981-14-6835-3

Published by Bentham Science Publishers Pte. Ltd. Singapore. All Rights Reserved.

need for a court order if at any point you breach any terms of this License Agreement. In no event will any delay or failure by Bentham Science Publishers in enforcing your compliance with this License Agreement constitute a waiver of any of its rights.

3. You acknowledge that you have read this License Agreement, and agree to be bound by its terms and conditions. To the extent that any other terms and conditions presented on any website of Bentham Science Publishers conflict with, or are inconsistent with, the terms and conditions set out in this License Agreement, you acknowledge that the terms and conditions set out in this License Agreement shall prevail.

Bentham Science Publishers Pte. Ltd.
80 Robinson Road #02-00
Singapore 068898
Singapore
Email: subscriptions@benthamscience.net

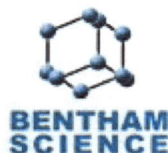

BENTHAM SCIENCE

CONTENTS

PREFACE

Civilizations throughout human history have benefited from the taste, aroma, and benefits of spices and culinary herbs. They contain among the most valued natural products for their culinary and recreational uses and medicinal properties. Many of them have become integral parts of traditional systems of medicine. In recent decades they have been the focus of extensive scientific research. Their remarkable health benefits have been demonstrated through numerous phytochemical, pharmacological and clinical studies.

The 3rd volume of the book series entitled, *"Science of Spices and Culinary Herbs"* is a compilation of eight excellent review articles, presenting the latest developments in this exciting field of natural product sciences. They cover a whole range of topics, all relevant to the evidence based therapeutic, nutritional, and olfactory uses of common spices and herbs.

The review by Marcelino *et al* is focused on the anthelmintic properties of cinnamon (*Cinnamomom verum* J. Presil.). Various helminthes parasites are associated with a plethora of diseases in host plants, farm animals, and humans. Several gastrointestinal diseases are also caused by helminthes is humans. The authors have provided a comprehensive chapter covering the scientific studies on anthelmintic properties of cinnamon and uses in agriculture crops, livestock, and humans. More *at al* have contributed a chapter on the nutraceutical and other important biological properties of tamarind (*Tamarindus indica* L.), used globally as a fruit, and as a spice. The authors have presented the advances in phytochemistry and in clinical research on this globally important dietary plant. The next review by Oyetaya and Odeniyi is also focused on the nutritional and health promoting phytochemicals of tamarind. Turmeric (*Curcuma longa* Linn.) has been the focus of vigorous researches since the last several decades. Sukandar and Ayuningtyas have provided a comprehensive account of recent clinical studies conducted on various turmeric based formulations including its phytoconstituents. The review focuses on the importance of well-designed clinical trials and proper formulations in the context of turmeric based medications. Pimple *et al* have written a well referenced and well written chapter on culinary and perfumery properties of the famous herb oregano (*Origanum majorana* Linn.), focusing on its traditional uses, phytochemistry, and on its medicinal and perfumery importance. Soni *et al* discuss the medicinal constituents of black pepper (*Piper nigrum* L.), most important among which is piperine a pungent alkaloid. Preclinical pharmacological data supports the therapeutic potential of black pepper and its constituents. Coriander (*Coriandrum sativum* L.) is a herb of global significance. Upaganlawar *et al* have focused the recent work on therapeutic importance of this famous herb as well as its phytochemistry and pharmacognosy. Soni and Soni in the last chapter of this volume have reviewed recent work on the increasingly popular spice flax seed (*Linum usitatissimum* L.). Extensive studies on its nutritional and medicinal constituents followed by pharmacological and preclinical studies, have shown it to be a valuable functional food for physical and mental health.

We gratefully acknowledge scholarly contributions and timely submissions of their review articles by leading experts in this field. We also appreciate the diligent work of Ms. Fariya Zulfiqar (Manager Publications) and Mr. Mahmood Alam (Director Publications) at Bentham Science Publishers. We sincerely hope that this volume will greatly benefit the scientific community interested in the fascinating science of spices and herbs.

Atta-ur-Rahman, *FRS*   **M. Iqbal Choudhary & Sammer Yousuf**
Kings College   H.E.J. Research Institute of Chemistry
University of Cambridge   International Center for Chemical and Biological Sciences
Cambridge   University of Karachi
UK   Karachi, Pakistan

List of Contributors

Aishwarya T. Devi	Department of Biotechnology Sri Jayachamarajendra College of Engineering, JSS Science and Technology University, JSS Research Foundation, SJCE Campus, Manasagangothri, Mysore - 570 006, Karnataka, India
Aman Upaganlawar	SNJB's SSDJ College of Pharmacy, Neminagar, Chandwad 423 101, India
Amrita M. Kulkarni	P. E. Society's Modern College of Pharmacy, Yamunanagar, Nigdi-411044, Pune, India
Anirudh Gururaj Patil	School of Basic and Applied Sciences, Department of Biological Sciences, Dayananda Sagar University, Shavige Malleshwara Hills, Kumaraswamy Layout, Bengaluru - 560 111, Karnataka, India
Ashish Singhai	Faculty of Pharmacy, VNS Group of Institutions, Bhopal 462044, India
Benjamín Nogueda-Torres	Escuela Nacional de Ciencias Biológicas, Instituto Politécnico Nacional. Prolongación de Carpio y Plan de Ayala s/n, Miguel Hidalgo, Santo Tomás, 11340 Ciudad de, México
Bhushan P. Pimple	P. E. Society's Modern College of Pharmacy, Yamunanagar, Nigdi-411044, Pune, India
Blanca Aguilar-Figueroa	Escuela Nacional de Ciencias Biológicas, Instituto Politécnico Nacional. Prolongación de Carpio y Plan de Ayala s/n, Miguel Hidalgo, Santo Tomás, 11340 Ciudad de, México
Blanca E. Álvarez-Fernández	Facultad de Ciencias Químico Biológicas de la Universidad Autónoma de Guerrero, Lázaro Cárdenas, S/N. Ciudad Universitaria, Chilpancingo, Guerrero, C.P. 39090, México
Dhyan K. Ayuningtyas	Department of Pharmacology and Clinical Pharmacy, School of Pharmacy, Bandung Institute of Technology, Bandung, Indonesia
Elin Y. Sukandar	Department of Pharmacology and Clinical Pharmacy, School of Pharmacy, Bandung Institute of Technology, Bandung, Indonesia
Farhan Zameer	School of Basic and Applied Sciences, Department of Biological Sciences, Dayananda Sagar University, Shavige Malleshwara Hills, Kumaraswamy Layout, Bengaluru - 560 111, Karnataka, India
F. Lucy Oyetayo	Department of Biochemistry, Ekiti State University, Ado-Ekiti, Ekiti State, Nigeria
Gabriela Oropeza-Guzman	Escuela Nacional de Ciencias Biológicas, Instituto Politécnico Nacional. Prolongación de Carpio y Plan de Ayala s/n, Miguel Hidalgo, Santo Tomás, 11340 Ciudad de, México
Gloria Sarahi Castañeda-Ramirez	Centro Nacional de Investigación Disciplinaria en Salud Animal e Inocuidad, INIFAP, Km 11 Carretera Federal Cuernavaca-Cuautla, No. 8534, Col. Progreso, Jiutepec, Morelos, CP 62550, México
Gloria Ivonne Hernández-Bolio	Departamento de Recursos del Mar, Centro de Investigación y de Estudios Avanzados del Instituto Politécnico Nacional, Unidad Mérida, México
Gonzalo Silva-Aguayo	Departamento de Producción Vegetal, Facultad de Agronomía, Universidad de Concepción, Vicente Méndez 595, Chillán, Chile

Javier Ventura-Cordero   School of Biological Sciences, Queen´s University Belfast, Chlorine Gardens, Belfast, BT95BL, UK

K. Muthucheliyan   School of Basic and Applied Sciences, Department of Biological Sciences, Dayananda Sagar University, Shavige Malleshwara Hills, Kumaraswamy Layout, Bengaluru - 560 111, Karnataka, India

Kounaina Khan   Department of Dravyaguna, JSS Ayurvedic Medical College, Lalithadripura, Mysuru - 570 028, Karnataka, India

Liliana Aguilar-Marcelino   Centro Nacional de Investigación Disciplinaria en Salud Animal e Inocuidad, INIFAP, Km 11 Carretera Federal Cuernavaca-Cuautla, No. 8534, Col. Progreso, Jiutepec, Morelos, CP 62550, México

Manuel Carrillo-Morales   Universidad Politécnica del Estado de Morelos, Boulevard Cuauhnáhuac #566, Col. Lomas del Texcal, C.P.62550, Jiutepec, Morelos, México

M.G. Avinash   Department of Studies in Microbiology, University of Mysore, Manasagangotri, Mysore – 570 006, Karnataka, India

M.N. Nagendra   Department of Biotechnology, Sri Jayachamarajendra College of Engineering, JSS Science and Technology University, JSS Research Foundation, SJCE Campus, Manasagangothri, Mysore - 570 006, Karnataka, India

Naveen Kumar Choudhary   Department of Pharmacognosy, Head of Herbal drug Research in B. R. Nahata College of Pharmacy, Mandsaur, M.P., India

Pankaj Satapathy   School of Basic and Applied Sciences, Department of Biological Sciences, Dayananda Sagar University, Shavige Malleshwara Hills, Kumaraswamy Layout, Bengaluru - 560 111, Karnataka, India

Priyanka Soni   Department of Pharmacognosy, Head of Herbal drug Research in B. R. Nahata College of Pharmacy, Mandsaur, M.P., India

Ruchita B. Bhor   P. E. Society's Modern College of Pharmacy, Yamunanagar, Nigdi-411044, Pune, India

S. Aishwarya   School of Basic and Applied Sciences, Department of Biological Sciences, Dayananda Sagar University, Shavige Malleshwara Hills, Kumaraswamy Layout, Bengaluru - 560 111, Karnataka, India

S.M. Veena   Department of Biotechnology, Sapthagiri College of Engineering, Bangalore - 560 057, India

Shubha Gopal   Department of Biotechnology, Sapthagiri College of Engineering, Bangalore - 560 057, India

Shubha Gopal   Department of Studies in Microbiology, University of Mysore, Manasagangotri, Mysore – 570 006, Karnataka, India

Shivaprasad Hudeda   Department of Dravyaguna, JSS Ayurvedic Medical College, Lalithadripura, Mysuru - 570 028, Karnataka, India

Sunil S. More   School of Basic and Applied Sciences, Department of Biological Sciences, Dayananda Sagar University, Shavige Malleshwara Hills, Kumaraswamy Layout, Bengaluru - 560 111, Karnataka, India

Vishal Soni   Department of Pharmacognosy, Head of Herbal drug Research in B. R. Nahata College of Pharmacy, Mandsaur, M.P., India

Vipin Dhote   Faculty of Pharmacy, VNS Group of Institutions, Bhopal 462044, India

Anthelmintic Properties of Cinnamon for the Control of Agricultural and Public Health Pests

Gloria Sarahi Castañeda-Ramirez[1], Javier Ventura-Cordero[2], Gloria Ivonne Hernández-Bolio[3], Gonzalo Silva-Aguayo[4], Manuel Carrillo-Morales[5], Gabriela Oropeza-Guzman[6], Blanca Aguilar-Figueroa[6], Benjamín Nogueda-Torres[6], Blanca E. Álvarez-Fernández[7] and Liliana Aguilar-Marcelino[1,*]

[1] *Centro Nacional de Investigación Disciplinaria en Salud Animal e Inocuidad, INIFAP, Km 11 Carretera Federal Cuernavaca-Cuautla, No. 8534, Col. Progreso, Jiutepec, Morelos, CP 62550, México*

[2] *School of Biological Sciences, Queen's University Belfast, Chlorine Gardens, Belfast, BT95BL, UK*

[3] *Departamento de Recursos del Mar, Centro de Investigación y de Estudios Avanzados del Instituto Politécnico Nacional, Unidad Mérida, México*

[4] *Departamento de Producción Vegetal, Facultad de Agronomía, Universidad de Concepción, Vicente Méndez 595, Chillán, Chile*

[5] *Universidad Politécnica del Estado de Morelos, Boulevard Cuauhnáhuac #566, Col. Lomas del Texcal, C.P.62550, Jiutepec, Morelos, México*

[6] *Escuela Nacional de Ciencias Biológicas, Instituto Politécnico Nacional. Prolongación de Carpio y Plan de Ayala s/n, Miguel Hidalgo, Santo Tomás, 11340 Ciudad de México, CDMX, México*

[7] *Facultad de Ciencias Químico Biológicas de la Universidad Autónoma de Guerrero, Av. Lázaro Cárdenas, S/N. Ciudad Universitaria, Chilpancingo, Guerrero, C.P. 39090, México*

Abstract: The most prevalent helminths are the gastrointestinal nematodes, such as the parasitic nematode *Haemonchus contortus* of sheep. Other economically important nematodes are phytoparasites, *Nacobbus aberrans* and *Meloidogyne incognita*, affecting more than 200 crops of plants and vegetables such as tomatoes, among others. Regarding the cestodes and *Hymenolepis nana* are the most prevalent worldwide. These helminths occur in warm temperate and dry geographical areas of developing countries with poor sanitary habits affecting mainly children between 2-8 years old. The conventional control is the use of anthelmintics (*e.g.* macrocyclic lactones, benzimidazoles and imidazoles) of synthetical origin; however, the misuse of these anthelmintics has led to a problem of chemical resistance worldwide; in addition,

* **Corresponding author L. Aguilar-Marcelino:** Centro Nacional de Investigación Disciplinaria en Salud Animal e Inocuidad, INIFAP, Km 11 Carretera Federal Cuernavaca-Cuautla, No. 8534, Col. Progreso, Jiutepec, Morelos, CP 62550, México; Tel: +52 777 319 28 60, Ext. 121; Fax: +52 777 31928 48, Ext. 129; E-mail: aguilar.liliana@inifap.gob.mx

Atta-ur-Rahman, M. Iqbal Choudhary & Sammer Yousuf (Eds.)

the residuality of these compounds in sheep byproducts, such as meat and milk, has caused a negative environmental impact. They also damage populations of beneficial organisms, such as the dung beetle, earthworms and nematophagous mites, among others. Hence, it is urgent and necessary to search for other integral, environmentally friendly, and sustainable control methods. The use of medicinal plants, mainly spices and culinary herbs, could be a sustainable alternative to control helminths that affect humans, plants and animals. This chapter presents an overview of the anthelmintic properties of cinnamon for sustainable helminth parasites control. This chapter is divided into several topics including 1) biology of cinnamon, 2) traditional and molecular taxonomic description of cinnamon, 3) metabolites reported in cinnamon, 4) uses of cinnamon as a condiment, 5) antiparasitic properties of cinnamon, 6) anthelmintic properties against agricultural pests, 7) anthelmintic properties against livestock pests and productive performance, 8) advances and perspectives of cinnamon in the control of anthelmintic properties, and 9) perspectives on the study of the anthelmintic properties of cinnamon.

Keywords: Anthelmintic properties, *Cinnamomum verum*, Culinary herbs, Spices, Soil-transmitted helminthes.

INTRODUCTION

The helminths are classified into flukes, cestodes, and nematodes [1, 2]. They inhabit intestinal and extraintestinal sites [3].

The control of parasitic helminths of agricultural and public health importance has been realized through the use of chemical products [4]; however, these products have been used indiscriminately and incorrectly, which has led to the emergence of resistance in the populations of these parasites to most of the commercially available active ingredients for the control of parasitic helminths of agricultural importance and public health [5].

Several plants have been used for medicinal applications and have been traditionally consumed as decoctions and infusions [6]. Mexico is a country that has a high medicinal plant diversity within this diversity of plants is cinnamon, which stands out mainly for use as a condiment in the preparation of various foods in the Mexican population [7].

The *Cinnamomum* genus consists of thousands of species that are distributed all over the world and is considered as one of the most important and popular spices used in cooking as well as traditional and modern medicines.

There are reports of beneficial bioactivity of this plant on health and against bacteria and viruses [8]. Based on the information described earlier in this chapter, it presents an overview of cinnamon's anthelmintic properties for agricultural and public health pest control.

BIOLOGY OF CINNAMON

The cinnamon tree has a long history. There exists evidence of its use since antiquity and we can find it in different texts. The first reported medical uses were documented in Egypt [9]. The cinnamon trees were initially found in Sri Lanka (Ceilan) in the 16th century, although, they are originally from India. Subsequently, they were imported to Europe and later cultivated in other parts of the world [10].

The name cinnamon corresponds to several species of the genus *Cinnamomum*. Nearly 250 species of this genus of trees and shrubs have been reported. Despite this large variety of species, only four are used for commercial purposes. These are *Cinnamomum zeylanicum* (Ceylon), *C. cassia* (Cassia), *C. loureirii* (Saigon) and *C. burmannii* (Korintje cinnamon) [11].

The cinnamon is a tree of 10 to 15 meters high, its leaves are perennial, and it is characterized by its leaves and bark, which are very aromatic. The leaves have a length of 7 to 25 cm and are opposite, their petiole is 1-2 cm long, green, oval (5-25 cm x 3-10 cm), leathery, with three prominent and shiny nerves. When the leaves are young, they present a reddish colour. The fruit is ovoid drupes of 12.5cm with only one seed inside, being mature in six months. Its flowers are hermaphrodite, small (from 3 mm to 6 mm length) and are presented in bunches. They can be either white or yellow and can be found mainly in January. The bark of this tree is rough and thick (10 mm) and mostly used as a species. It can be gray or brown, while the stem is woody. On the bark, there are strips of 50 cm long [12]; this tree is used in the food industry due to its flavor, the younger the branches, the better the quality [14, 13]. From the bark, perfumes, aromatics, and tea, among other things, are prepared [15] (Fig. **1**).

Cinnamon trees can tolerate different climatic conditions, mainly preferring a warm and humid climate [16]. Mainly the trees prefer a warm and humid climate [17]. The tree flourishes in places with an annular rainfall of 1500-2500 mm at 27 degrees [18]. According to Krishnamoorthy [19], they reported that the Navashree (SL63) and Nithyashree (IN 189) varieties produce 55.6 kg and 54.2 kg of bark/hectare/per year. It is very important to consider regeneration capacity and yield.

From the ecological point of view, it is known that *C. verum* can become invasive and may affect the regeneration in poorly-nutrient tropical secondary forests; this is due to the dense topsoil sphere of *C. verum* [20].

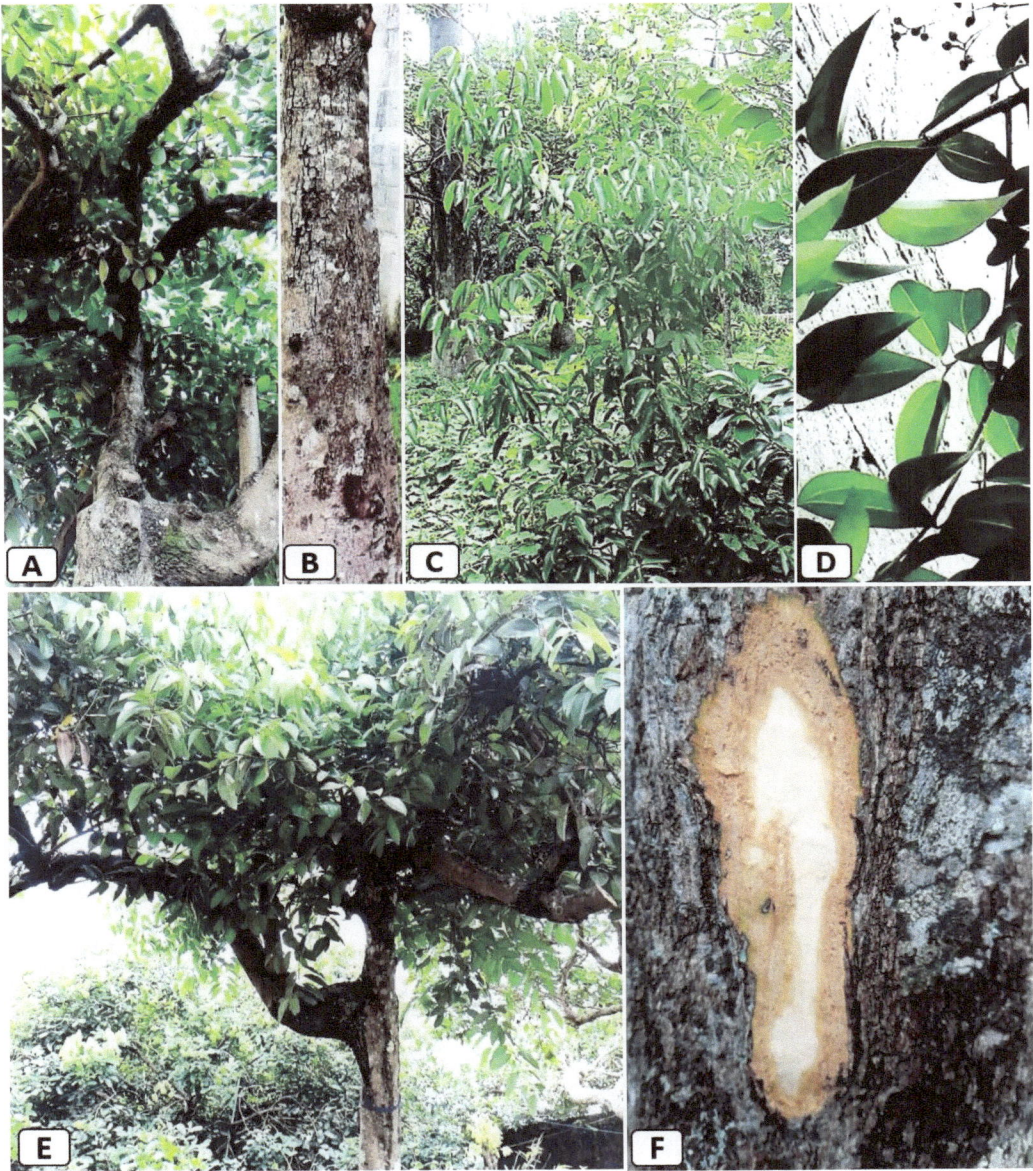

Fig. (1). Cinnamon tree, Southern Chiapas, Mexico (Courtesy. Dr Guillermo López-Guillén and M.C Stephania Colmenares-Cruz). **A)** adult tree, **B)** cinnamon tree bark, **C)** young tree, **D)** cinnamon tree leaves and fruit, **E)** Forms that the tree can acquire and **F)** cutting in the tree bark.

TRADITIONAL AND MOLECULAR TAXONOMIC DESCRIPTION OF CINNAMON

Traditional Taxonomy

For traditional taxonomic identification, measurements and observation of the following tree parts have been used: shape of the trunk, the bark, the shape and color of the leaves, the distribution of the branches, if they have thorns, the flowers, and the characteristics of the fruits.

There are about 250 species of the genus *Cinnamomum*. This genus belongs to the family Lauraceae, which includes 2,850 species, among them *Persea americana* and *Laurus nobilis* [21]. Particularly, the cinnamon tree was first described by the chemist, botanist Jan Svatopluk Presl in 1825 "*Cinnamomum verum*".

The word *Cinnamomum* comes from the Greek word *Kinnamon* or *Kinnamomon* which means sweet wood, in turn, this term comes from the Hebrew word *quinamom* with the same meaning. On the other hand, the word cinnamon comes from the French word *cannelle,* which means cane or tube. Below is the taxonomy of *Cinnamomum*.

    Kingdom: Plantae
    Division: Magnoliophyta
    Class: Magnoliopside
    Order: Laurals
    Family: Lauraceae
    Genus: *Cinnamomum*

Molecular Taxonomy

Currently, the genome of a species of *Cinnamomum* has been reported; this species was *Cinnamomum kanehirae,* also known as camphor tree, in turn, it is also the first member sequenced Magnoliidae (Laural, Magnoliales, Canellales and Piperales). The genome size was approximately 823.7 ± 58.2 Mb / 1 C [21]. On the other hand, *Cinnamomum verum* Presl. is synonymous with *C. zeylanicum* Bl. with a chromosome number of $2n = 24$. The genome of an organism comprises the entirety of its DNA.

The molecular biology has been used to identify species and through phylogenetic trees to understand the similarity of species between different parts of the world [22]. The traditional identification of *Cinnamomum* species has been based on expert botanical classification based on morphology or histological microscopy;

however, identification based on morphological characteristics is difficult due to morphological similarities between species.

A work reported the identification of species with molecular techniques: samples were collected from seven species of *Cinnamomum* (*C. cassia, C. verum, C. burmanni, C. pauciflorum, C. iners, C. japonicum* and *C. camphora*). They found differences between the species by means of the sequences [23].

However, there is a wide variety of methodologies for the molecular taxonomic identification of plants, even more so in specialized laboratories with modified plant lineages. One could say that ideally, for sequences, it should allow precise identification. On the other hand, when selecting a location to obtain the sequence, universal application and maximum rates of sequence divergence are needed, which cause some variants [24, 25].

One study determined which sites could maximize species identification when combined as a code based on DNA sequences. It indicated that a variety of DNA loci have been suggested for plants, including encoding genes and non-coding spacers in the nuclear and plastidic genomes [26].

METABOLITES REPORTED IN CINNAMON

The *Cinnamomum* genus is characterized by the presence of a wide variety of odor and flavoring compunds that are present in almost the whole plant. These metabolites give their particular properties to the different species; however, additional non-volatile compounds are interesting since they explains the diverse bioactivities reported from plants belonging to this genus. Examples of these compounds are presented in this section.

Volatiles

Undoubtedly, owing to their flavoring, cosmetic, and gastronomic importance, the volatiles are the most studied components of the *Cinnamomum* species. Their profile differs according to the diverse parts of the plant utilized to extract the oil, commonly made by steam distillation. Most of the studies use gas chromatography coupled to mass spectrometry since it simplifies the detection process, and particularly, the identification of the low mass metabolites. In the following part, the main components of the oils extracted from different plant parts are described.

Leaves

A total of 41 compounds have been reported from the leaves oil, with eugenol (**1**) being the major constituent (about 70% of total volatiles). Additional components of quantitative importance are the terpenes caryophyllene and linalool, as well as the aromatic ester benzyl benzoate [27]. However, the method of extraction can affect the content of the major components, for instance, the hydrodistillation of the *C. zeylanicum* leaves led to an oil containing 85.7% linalool (**2**), followed by eugenol (3.1%) and *β*-caryophyllene (2.4%) [28]. The profile of compounds present in the essential oil also varies regarding the species of *Cinnamomum* studied: the hydrodistillation of five cinnamon species reported *trans*-cinnamaldehyde (**3**) as present in all the extracts and as a major component of *C. cassia* and *C. burmannii*. In addition, 3-methoxy-1,2-propanediol (**4**) was the main volatile compound *C. cassia* leaf, while eugenol of *C. zeylanicum*, *C. pauciflorum* and *C. burmannii* leaves, and 5-(2-propenyl)-1,3-benzodioxole (**5**) of *C. tamala* leaf were also the main components [29].

Bark

The principal constituents of *Cinnamomum* bark oil are cinnamaldehyde (**3**) (60-70%) and cinnamyl acetate (8-10%), along with additional minor components as cineole, linalool, caryophyllene and eugenol [27]. Besides the presence of common mono and sesquiterpenes, aromatic compounds such as benzaldehyde, methyl chavicol, hydrocinnamaldehyde, 2-phenetyl alcohol, 2-phenylpropylacetate, and coumarin have been identified in the bark oil additional minor components also such as cineole, linalool, caryophyllene and eugenol [27]. Furthermore, two new pentacyclic terpenoids with a unique structure, named cinnzeylanine (**6**) and cinnzeylanol (**7**) were isolated from the dried bark of *C. zeylanicum* [30].

Root bark

The monoterpene camphor (**8**) is the major component of root bark oil (56%), while other constituents such as cineole, α-terpineol, α-pinene, and limonene are also of great importance [27].

Fruit Stalks

Approximately 27 compounds have been reported from the fruit stalks. The major volatiles found in this plant part after steam distillation are, the (*E*)-cinnamyl acetate (**9**) (36.6%) and (*E*)-caryophyllene (**10**) (22.4%). Additional compounds of importance are sesquiterpene alcohols τ-cadinol and ledol (4.9% and 2.5%, respectively) [31].

Fruits

More than 30 components represent 94% of the oil from *C. zeylanicum* fruit. The *trans*-cinnamyl acetate (**9**) and *β*-caryophyllene (**10**) were found to be the major compounds, accompanied by 3-phenylpropyl acetate, cinnamyl alcohol, cis and *trans*-cinnamaldehyde. The sesquiterpenes *α*-humulene, *α*-copaene, *δ* and *γ*-cadinene, and germacrene B, are also present in abundance [32].

Chart 1

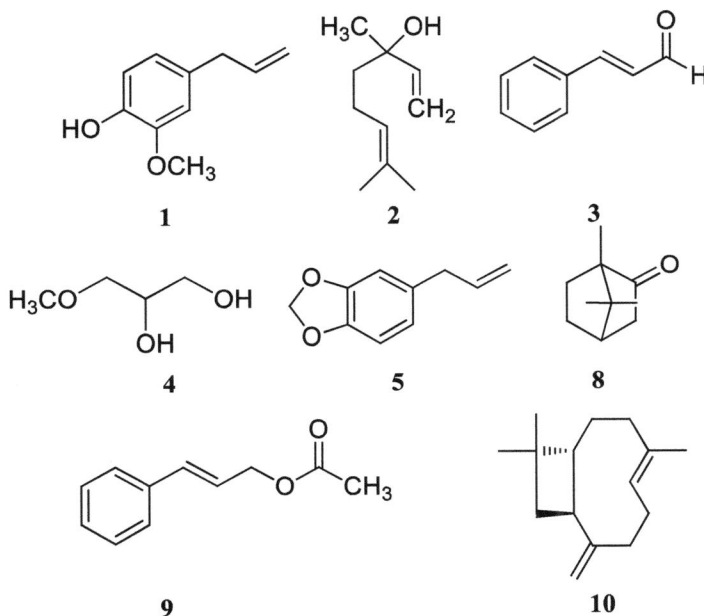

Chart 2

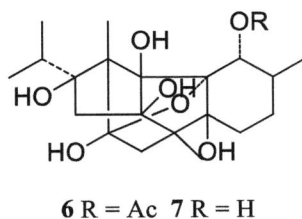

6 R = Ac 7 R = H

Phenolics

Simple Phenolics

The *Cinnamomum* species, as almost every type of plant, possess common phenolic compounds that have been identified mainly from the bark. Flavanols as catechin (**11**) and epicatechin (**12**), together with phenylpropanoids as the caffeic (**13**), ferulic (**14**), *p*-coumaric (**15**), protocatechuic (**16**), and vanillic (**17**) acids, have been successfully extracted using subcritical water extraction given the high polarity. The extraction of less polar phenolics, which are also the major flavoring components, such as cinnamaldehyde (**3**), cinnamic acid (**18**), cinnamyl alcohol (**19**), and coumarin (**20**), is favored by maceration with methanol [33]. The cinnamon fruits were also investigated for antioxidant activity, resulting in the isolation of five phenolic compounds: protocatechuic acid (**16**), cinnamtannin B-1, urolignoside (**21**), rutin (**22**), and quercetin rhamnopyranoside (**23**) [34]. In addition, a new lignin, cinnamophilin (**24**), along with three known compounds, *meso*-dihydroguaiaretic acid (**25**), (+)-guaiacin (**26**), and vanillic acid (**17**), was isolated from the root of *C. philippinense* [35].

Chart 3

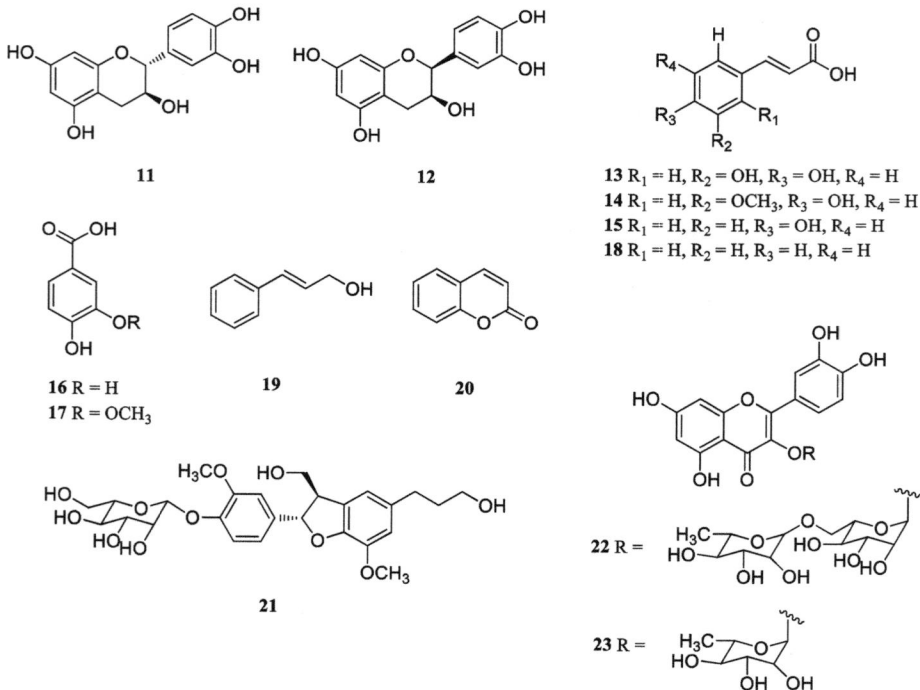

11

12

13 R_1 = H, R_2 = OH, R_3 = OH, R_4 = H
14 R_1 = H, R_2 = OCH$_3$, R_3 = OH, R_4 = H
15 R_1 = H, R_2 = H, R_3 = OH, R_4 = H
18 R_1 = H, R_2 = H, R_3 = H, R_4 = H

16 R = H
17 R = OCH$_3$

19

20

21

22 R =

23 R =

Chart 4

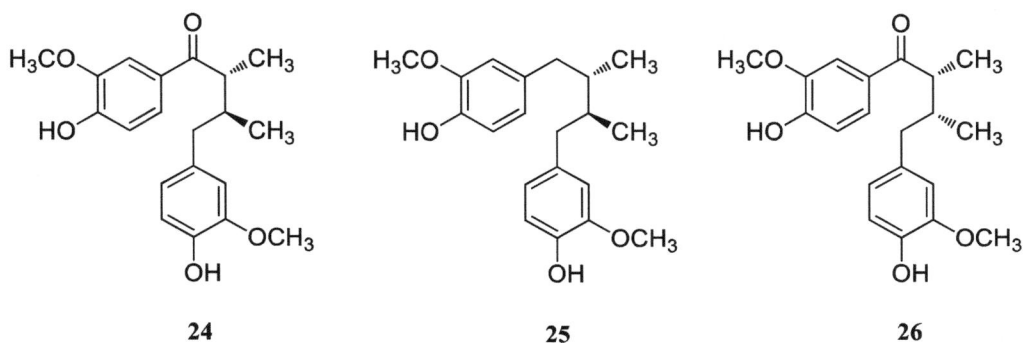

24 25 26

Polyphenols

Although less studied, cinnamon is a rich source of polyphenolic compounds. For instance, water-soluble polymers from cinnamon were isolated and characterized, indicating that they are A-type (containing C4→C8 carbon and C2→O7 ether bonds between the terminal and middle units of the trimer) [36]. Similarly, procyanidin B2 (**27**) was identified from the aqueous extract of cinnamon bark, as well as common phenolics [37]. Extracts prepared from bark of other species of *Cinnamomum* such as *C. tamala* and *C. cassia*, led to the isolation of six compounds namely procyanidin B2 (**27**), (-)-epicatechin (**12**), the trimers cinnamtannin B1 (**28**), procyanidin C1 (**29**), and cinnamtannin D1 (**30**), and the tetramer parameritannin A1 [38].

Alkaloids

The alkaloids of the *Cinnamomum* genus have been explored from less-studied species and diverse plant parts. The isolated compounds belong to different types of alkaloids. For instance, the methanolic extraction of the *C. philippinense* roots led to the isolation of six alkaloids including a new pyridine, 2-(4--hydroxypyridin-3'-yl)-acetic acid (**31**), an amide, cinnaretamine (**32**), a benzylisoquinoline, crykonisine (**33**), an isoquinolone, corydaldine (**34**), a proaporphine, glaziovine (**35**), and an aporphine, zenkerine (**36**) [39]. Additionally, another new pyridine, cinnapine (**37**), was reported from the root extract of *C. philippinense* [40].

Chart 5

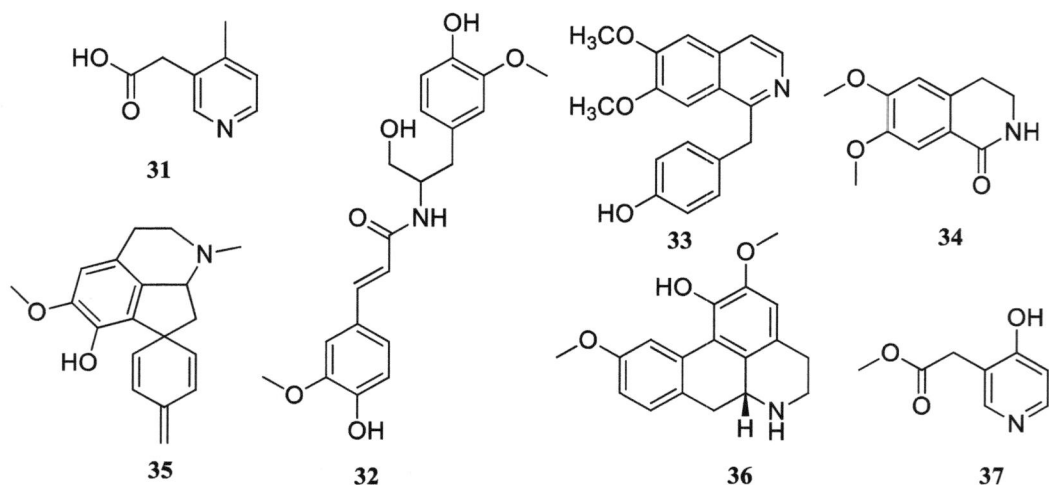

From the bark of *C. mollissimum,* five aporphine alkaloids were isolated. The crude alkaloid extraction and characterization led to the identification of *N*-methyl-1,2,10-trimethoxyaporphine (**38**), *N*-methylhernagine (**39**), *N*-methylhernovine (**40**), hernagine (**41**), and hernovine (**42**) [41]. In a similar way, the major alkaloids from the bark of *C. camphora* were identified as the benzylisoquinolines norcinnamolaurine (a new compound) (**43**), (---cinnamolaurine (**44**), and (+)-reticuline (**45**), together with the aporphine (+)-corydine (**46**) [42].

Chart 6

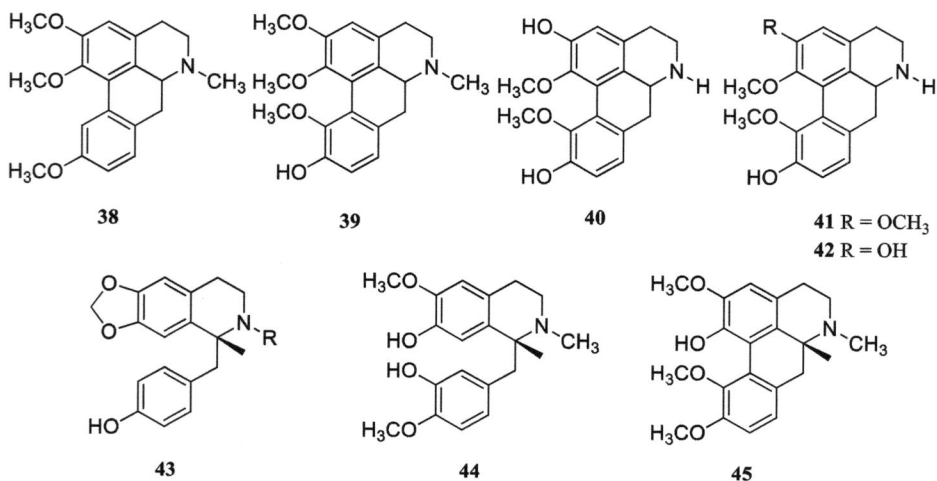

Additional phytochemical screening of different *Cinnamomum* species reported the presence of further compounds, namely saponins, flavonoids, *etc.*; however, to our knowledge, none of these metabolites have been isolated or identified.

USES OF CINNAMON AS A CONDIMENT

Cinnamon has been used as a condiment and flavoring in food worldwide, in some cultures is important consumption of this spice for its medicinal and nutritional properties. Based on information reported by Codex Alimentarius, it has reported that by-products that are classified as spices, soups, *etc.*, add other substances to improve their flavor and aroma [43, 44].

Cinnamon has a mild or delicate aroma and flavour (Cinnamomum spp.). In addition, it possesses several nutritional properties, in particular it is an important source of iron, calcium and a high percentage of dietary fiber; a source of manganese has also been reported to be present in this condiment. Other important nutrients are fatty acids, amino acids and carbohydrates [45 - 47]. The bark of the cinnamon tree is consumed as infusions, marinades or tea.

One of the applications of cinnamon is as a preservative for various foods and especially for inhibiting the growth of pathogenic populations. The compounds that have been reported in cinnamon oil are mainly: cinnamyl alcohol and eugenol, among others [48].

Another medicinal use is the use of cinnamon to treat and relieve toothache caused by varicose veins pathogens such as bacteria. In some cultures cinnamon is used directly from the bark of the tree to improve digestion [49]. Currently, several companies use cinnamon because of its versatility, as an additive to improve the flavors and aromas of the products they make, thus taking advantage of the aroma of cinnamon [50].

ANTIPARASITIC PROPERTIES OF CINNAMON

Antiprotozoal Properties of Cinnamon

There exist a number of general cellular targets that can mediate cytotoxicity in human cells but also in parasites [51]. The essential oil of cinnamon or its components has currently been shown to have inhibitory activity on protozoa such as *Plasmodium falciparum* [52, 53] piroplasms [8] and *Trypanosoma cruzi* [54].

Through a phase, I clinical trial, the efficacy and safety of *C. zeylanicum* were demonstrated, showing that, after three months of ingesting capsules with powdered bark of *C. zeylanicum,* the individuals did not show significant side effects and toxicity [55].

Activity against *Plasmodium falciparum*

Medicines that have been used clinically and that have one of these two ways of action include chloroquine, amodiaquine, quinine, sulfadoxine-pyrimethamine, artemisinin derivatives (predominantly artemether and artesunate), and lumefantrine [56 - 58].

Nkanwen *et al.,* (2013) made extracts with CH_2Cl_2/MeOH (1: 1) from the stem bark of *C. zeylanicum*; these extracts were fractionated and purified. Obtaining six compounds: transcinamic anhydride (1), ferulic acid (2), (E) p-hydroxycinnamic acid (3), clovanodiol (4), squalene (5) and α-bisabolene (6) [59]. *In vitro,* compounds 1, 5, and 6 exhibited inhibitory activity against the *P. falciparum* enzyme enoyl-ACP reductase (PfENR) at 17.0, 24.3, and 33.3%, respectively [59].

Parvazi [53] using ^{1}H-NMR spectroscopy reported the *in vitro* effect of the aqueous extract of *Cinnamomum cassia* against the metabolism of *P. falciparum.* The bioactive metabolites were identified as succinic acid, glutathione, L-aspartic acid, beta-alanine and 2-methylbutyrylglycine.

Activity against Pyroplasmas

The best treatment of babesiosis in humans is the combination of atovaquone with azithromycin due to its low side effects [60]. Despite this benefit, some human cases showed resistance to the combination [8].

Viability tests carried out by Batiha [8] showed the inhibitory effect *in vitro* and *in vivo* of *C. verum* acetone extract (AECV) and *C. verum* ethyl acetate extract (EAECV) against piroplasm parasites.

Activity against *Trypanosoma cruzi*

Chagas disease affects several millions of people in Latin America and is spreading beyond its classical limits due to the migration of infected vectors from hosts and insects, HIV coinfection and blood transfusion [61].

Several essential oils, or their constituents, have recently been shown to have inhibitory activity against *Trypanosoma cruzi.* Azeredo [54] evaluated the effect of the following essential oils (EO) against epimastigote forms of *T. cruzi: Cinnamomum verum* (formerly *Cinnamomum zeylanicum; Lauraceae; cinnamon).*

Among the essential oils analyzed, *C. verum* showed the highest activity against *T. cruzi* epimastigotes.

Activity against *Schistosoma japonicum*

Schistosomiasis by *S. japonicum* is considered as an economic and public health concern in China, the Philippines and Indonesia. Linalool is a major component in leaf extracts of *Cinnamomum camphora*. After exposure to linalool, a damage to the gills and hepatopancreas of the snails was observed with a cercaricidal activity. In addition, linalool markedly reduced the recovered schistosomulum from mouse skin after challenge infection [62].

ANTHELMINTIC PROPERTIES AGAINST AGRICULTURAL PESTS

Insecticidal Activity

Botanical insecticides were the first pest control strategies, but when synthetic insecticides appeared, they were "forgotten". For many decades, synthetic insecticides have been almost the only pest control alternative mainly for effectiveness and easy to use. However, problems like residues, pest resistance and environmental pollution have reconsidered the use of biopesticides. The classical botanical insecticides are the neem (*Azadirachta indica* J.; Meliaceae), nicotine sulfate (*Nicotiana tabacum* L.; Solanaceae), and rotenone, obtained from *Derris*, *Lonchocarpus*, and *Tephrosia* species. However, recently, in different countries, much research is taking place on new plants with insecticidal activity. One of these plants is *Cinnamomum* genus, particularly its essential oil.

Mode of Action

The presence of phenolic and volatile compounds in cinnamon essential oil provides the characteristic flavor and aroma to this spice. The main compounds detected in different varieties of cinnamon are cinnamaldeyde, cinnamyl-acetate, eugenol, linalool, and camphor among others [63 - 66]. All of these compounds have shown insecticidal activity against several agricultural, urban, veterinary and human health pests. According to Enan [67] and Rattan [68], the mode of action of essential oils is not fully elucidated, but all signals indicated neurotoxicity, however, depending on the components and concentrations, the site of action may vary. According to Rattan [68], the mechanisms affected by essential oils are the cholinergic system, GABA system, mitochondrial system and octopaminergic system. Enan [67] assessed the activity of eugenol, one of the principal components of cinnamon essential oil, concluding that the octopaminergic system mediated the insecticidal activity of eugenol. Tong and Coats [69] working on housefly and the monoterpenoids eugenol, linalool and cinnamic acid, concluded that monoterpenoid structure is strongly involved in binding activities to the housefly GABA receptors. According to Jain [65], a concentration of 53.2 µg mL-1 of an extract of *C. zeylanicum* demonstrated a potent inhibition of acetylcholinesterase. Also, the cinnamon essential oil has reported additional modes of action. In lepidopteran larvae, Gershenzon and Dudareva [70], indicated that terpenes block the stimulatory effects of glucose and inositol on chemosensory receptor cells located on the mouthparts, and they could act on receptors in other ways. Other authors report that cinnamon essential oil reduces the oviposition and adult emergence of *Callosobruchus maculatus* [71, 72], decreases respiratory rate, accelerates offspring and delays the emergence of females compared to males of *Sitophilus zeamais* [73].

Agricultural Pests

Control of agricultural pests using essential oils is usually focused on stored grain pests and scientific literature has many relevant publications. The genus *Sitophilus* spp is one of the most studied. The first results of *Cinnamomun* spp. as a grain protector against *Sitophilus* genus were obtained with powdered *C. zeylanicum* as Ashouri [74], where the concentration of 5.0% (w/w) showed the highest toxicity against adults of *S. granaries but* did not obtain 100% elimination of insects. Another study against the same insect [75], concluded that *C. zeylanicum* essential oil and their terpenoids are toxic and repellent. According to these authors, the terpenoid eugenol is the one with the highest toxicity to the insect, reducing the respiratory rate and mobility on a terpenoid treated surface. About *S. oryzae,* Kim [76] assessed an extract of *C. sieboldi* root bark and essential oil of *C. cassia* bark. The extract caused a 100% mortality at two days after treatments and the oil exhibited the same result as a fumigant. Lee [77] confirmed the fumigant activity against *S. oryzae* of four essential oils from bark and leaves of *Cinnamomun* showing an LD_{50} = 0.0003 mg cm^2, very similar to the synthetic insecticide Dichlorvos, with an LD_{50} = 0.00025 mg cm^2. Extracts of *Cinnamomun* [78], at three hours of exposure 3 mL dish^{-1} caused 90-99% mortality, although this result was dependent on exposure time and concentration. Finally, *S. zeamais* may be the most studied cinnamon essential oil that has a long history as an insecticide against this insect. Li [79] studied the toxicity of cinnamon oil, showing high repellent and fumigant activity against adults of *S. zeamais*. Haddi [73] reported an LC_{95} = 3.47 µl cm^{-2} and a significantly reduced respiratory rate in insects treated with the essential oil of *C. zeylanicum*.

Other relevant pests of stored seeds are the cowpea weevil (*Callosobruchus maculatus* (F.); Coleoptera: Bruchidae)) and the pulse beetle (*Callosobruchus chinensis* L.), both key pests of stored legumes. Brari and Thakur [80] assessed the contact and fumigant toxicity of *C. zeylanicum* against *C. maculatus;* they obtained rates of 98 and 80% mortality after 24 hours of treatment with a concentration of 1.2 mg cm^{-2}. Regarding the fumigant activity, the results were similar. Furthermore, Jumbo [81] indicated that the same essential oil exhibited insecticidal activity similar to the synthetic pyrethroid deltamethrin against *C. maculatus*. Islam [71] assessed the toxic activity of *C. aromaticum* against *C. maculatus*, reporting an LD$_{50}$ of 27.56 and 23.16 µg cm^{-2} after 24 and 48 h of exposure, respectively. Kim [76] evaluated an extract of *C. cassia* bark in a concentration of 3.5 mg cm^{-2}, which resulted in potent insecticidal activity against the pulse beetle, *C. chinensis*. Another member of the Bruchidae family is the bean weevil (*Acanthoscelides obtectus* Say), which causes severe post-harvest losses in the common bean (*Phaseolus vulgaris* L.). Jumbo [72] found insecticidal and repellent effect against adults of *A. obtectus* using the essential oil of *C. zeylanicum*.

The Indian meal moth (*Plodia interpunctella* Hübner; Lepidoptera: Pyralidae) and the lesser grain borer (*Rhyzoperta dominica* (F.): Coleoptera: Bostrychidae) are insects associated to stored cereals too, and the cinnamon has also been used for their control. Ashouri [74] assessed the powder of *C. zeylanicum* at 5.0% (w/w) against *R. dominica*, which exhibited significant toxicity on adults but did not cause 100% mortality. Against *P. interpunctella*, Jo [82], developed an anti-insect polymer strip using essential oil of *C. zeylanicum* in polyvinyl alcohol showing a 63% of mortality for fumigation at 120 h and effective repellency.

The essential oil of *C. cassia* was assessed by Park [83] against the agricultural pests' diamondback moth (*Plutella xylostella* L.: Plutellidae), green peach aphid (*Myzus persicae* Sulzer; Hemiptera: Aphidae), and two-spotted spider mite (*Tetranychus urticae* Koch; Acari: Tetranychidae). These authors concluded that *C. cassia* essential oil could be an effective natural acaricide and insecticide against these insect pests.

The lepidopterous moths are very important pests, and two examples of them are the cotton leafworm (*Spodoptera litura* Fabricius; Noctuidae) and the tomato pinworm (*Tuta absoluta* (Meyrick); Gelechiidae). The essential oil of cinnamon showed to increase rotenone toxicity when tested as a mixture against *S. litura* [79]. In tomato pinworm, *C. zeylanicum* essential oil was able to induce 100% of larvae mortality within four hours of exposure.

Finally, two additional agricultural pests in which cinnamon essential oil has been evaluated are the citrus flatid planthopper (*Metcalfa pruinosa* Say; Hemiptera: Flatidae) and the oak nut weevil (*Mechoris ursulus* Roelofs; Coleoptera: Attelabidae). In the case of *M. ursulus*, Park [84] assessed individually the main components of *C. cassia* essential oil concluding that the *trans*-cinnamaldehyde, eugenol and salicylaldehyde showed mortalities above 80%. The citrus flatid planthopper was examined using a direct-contact application bioassay exhibiting similar results to *M. ursulus,* as the most toxic constituents of essential oil were the hydroxy-cinnamic acid and eugenol [63].

Urban and Human Health Pests

An urban pest is defined as an organism that hinders with human activities. Urban pests are flies, mosquitoes, cockroaches, lice, fleas, ants, bed bugs and termites, among others. Several of these insects are vectors of pathogens that affect human health. Hence, using synthetic insecticides in the urban environment is very dangerous, particularly to children, pregnant women, and elders. For this reason, natural insecticides, as essentials oils represent an alternative. In the case of cinnamon, Ahmad [85] studied the repellent activity of *C. zeylanicum* essential oil against the domiciliary cockroach (*Periplaneta americana* L.; Dictyoptera: Blattellidae) obtaining 100% repellency with a concetration of 12 ppm. In a different study, Phillips [86] assessed the topical toxicity of two main constituents of *C. zeylanicum* essential oil, *trans*-cinnamaldehyde and eugenol, against the German cockroach (*Blatella germanica* L.; Dictyoptera: Blattellidae), showing the trans-cinnamaldehyde as the one with the highest toxicity against adult females, large nymphs, and small nymphs with LD_{50} values of 0.19, 0.12, and 0.04 mg per cockroach, respectively. Another urban pest with worldwide distribution and relevance is the housefly (*Musca domestica* L.; Diptera: Muscidae), an insect with many cases of resistance to synthetic insecticides. Sinthusiri and Soonwera [87] evaluated the effect of 20 essential oils against *M. Domestica,* demonstrating a knockdown effect of a 10% *C. verum* essential oil at 24 hours of 44.3 min and an $LC_{50} = 7.48\%$. Boito [88] assessed the effect of essential oil of *C. zeylanicum* against adult and larvae of *M. domestica* showing mortality of 100% after 90 minutes of exposure. At the same time, Khater and Geden [89] concluded that the essential oil of *C. zeylanicum* exhibited mortality of 100% and a strong repellency.

The ants are insects that people rarely perceive as a pest, but rather as beneficial. However, many species are considered urban pests. Kasim [90] evaluated the essential oil of *C. cassia* against ants), concluding that the essential oil has positive insecticidal and repellent activity. One of the most dangerous ants to humans is the red imported fire ant (*Solenopsis invicta* Buren; Hymenoptera: Formicidae) and, usually, insecticidal treatments are applied to soil for their control. Huang [91] tested a mixing of the soil with cinnamaldehyde and eugenol, two of the most abundant components discovering that the highest concentration is located at 5-10 cm, and that at this depth, it results in 100% mortality and a repellency of 96.3%. Another species of ant in which essential oils have been used is odors house ant (*Tapinoma sessile* Say; Hymenoptera: Formicidae) and according to Mutalib [92] *C. zeylanicum* essential oil is an effective repellent and insecticide against *T. sessile*.

Finally, the mosquitoes show a situation very similar to houseflies because there are many reports of insecticide resistance, so alternatives of control are necessary. Benelli [93] assessed the essential oil of *C. verum* against the Southern house mosquito (*Culex quinquefasciatus* Say; Diptera: Culicidae) obtaining the highest toxicity against 4th instar larvae with a LC$_{50}$ = 40.7 µL^{-1}, reducing adult emergence and fertility too. Cheng [94] evaluated essential oil of leaves of *Cinnamomum osmophloeum* against *C. quinquefasciatus*, *Aedes albopictus* Skuse and *Armigeres subalbatus* Coquillett. Results of larvicidal tests demonstrated that the leaf essential oil had an excellent inhibitory effect against *A. albopictus* larvae. Other mosquito species assessed with cinnamon essential oil is *Anopheles gambiae sensu lato* by Thomas [95], showing larvicidal effect at concentration-dependent doses.

Veterinary Pests

The veterinary pest associated with pets and livestock has been a research topic, and the cinnamon esential oil has been evaluated against pests of veterinary importance too. Khater [96] assessed the toxicity of *C. zeylanicum* essential oil against the sheep blowfly (*Lucilia sericata* (Meigen); Diptera: Calliphoridae), concluding that a dose of 5.0% produces larval mortality of 95.56%. The poultry red mite (*Dermanyssus gallinae* De Geer; Acari: Dermanyssidae) is an haematophagous ectoparasite of domestic poultry, a possible vector of various poultry pathogens. Na [97] studied the fumigant toxicity of four cinnamon oils exhibiting a good fumigant activity with an LD$_{50}$ = 26.4 g cm$^{-2,}$ resulting in a similar activity to the synthetic insecticide Dichlorvos. Other veterinary pests are the Horn fly (*Haemotobia irritans* L.; Diptera: Muscidae) and the Cattle tick (*Rhicicephalus microplus* Canestrini; Ixodida: Ixodidae). In the case of *H. irritans,* Boito [88], using naturally infested cows, evaluated the free and nanoemulsion essential oil of *C. zeylanicum*. The results showed that cinnamon oil at 10%, and the nanoemulsion in a concentration of 5.0% were 100% effective as contact insecticide and repellent against *H. irritans*. Finally, Khater [98] investigated the louscicidal and repellent effects of *C. camphora* L. against the buffalo louse (*Haematopinus tuberculatus* Burmeister; Phthiraptera: Haematopinidae), showing that the number of lice infesting buffaloes significantly reduced after treatment with *C. camphora* essential oil.

ANTHELMINTIC PROPERTIES AGAINST LIVESTOCK PESTS

Parasites at a worldwide level are considered the most important threat to animal production, causing impairments in animal health, live weight gain, milk production, wool production, feed conversion, and other performance parameters. Therefore, currently, many alternatives are being investigated to develop new methods of anthelmintic (AH) biocontrol, for instance, plants, spices, by-products, functional feeds, pre and probiotics [99, 100].

Cinnamon (*Cinnamomum* spp.) has demonstrated *in vitro* and *in vivo* anthelmintic activity against several organisms in livestock (cattle, poultry, sheep, goats, swine). Different solvents to obtain specific plant secondary metabolites from *C. verum* have been tested to identify if cinnamon could be used as a biocontrol method in animal production.

In this section, we showed the AH effects of cinnamon including essential oils and extracts in livestock production. For example, indirect and direct activities in the host allowed animals to fight from gastrointestinal nematodes.

Cinnamaldehyde is the main metabolite extracted from cinnamon's bark essential oil. This compound showed the highest egg hatch inhibition using an *Haemonchus contortus* multi-resistant isolate. The lethal concentration to kill 50% eggs mortality was 0.018 mg/mL (0.017-0.019 confidence intervals) [101]. The latter is highlighted evidence considering the recent rise of gastrointestinal nematodes resistance to conventional anthelmintic in sheep and goats. However, more *in vivo* will be necessary to confirm the AH effect in small ruminants infected naturally with gastrointestinal nematodes.

Acetonic extracts obtained from cinnamon's bark showed a strong *in vitro* AH activity against *Ascaris suun*, *Trichuris suis*, and *Oesophagostomum dentatum*. The secondary metabolites involved in the effect against helminths were proanthocyanidins and trans-cinnamaldehyde [102]. The study evaluated the *in vivo* effect of cinnamon´s capsule in Danish Landrace/Yorkshire/Duroc pigs; however, they did not find a reduction in the number larval burdens of *A. suun*.

A mixture of cinnamaldehyde (5 mg/kg), carvacrol 3 (mg/kg), and *Capsicum oleoresin* (2 mg/kg) was offered to broiler chickens orally infected with 2.0×10^4 sporulated virulent oocysts of *Eimeria tenella*. The latter supplementation improved the immune system, increased body weight, and reduced the number of oocysts in chickens [103].

As we mentioned before, the cinnamaldehyde represented the highest compound from essential oils after the extraction of cinnamon bark. A commercial cinnamon essential oil was used to evaluate the *in vitro* acaricidal activity against unfed larvae of *Rhipicephalus* (*Boophilus*) *microplus* (Acari: Ixodidae). The study reported that the highest acaricidal effect against larvae was of the essential oil from cinnamon when compared with a mixture of clove and lemongrass essential oils [104].

Productive Performance

In this section, we show some effects of cinnamon on the productive performance of livestock.

The addition of cinnamon's extracts to goat milk could improve the antioxidant capacity, according to Setiyoningrum [105]. Also, the essential oils have shown an antimicrobial activity against *Klebsiella* spp in milk from cows, buffaloes, sheep, and goats [106]. On the other hand, cinnamon powder has been used to change the organoleptic characteristics of soft white cheese from goats. The latter was to improve the acceptance of consumers and because it is considered that secondary metabolites from spices delay the bacteria growth. No differences were reported in the chemical composition of cheese, although cheese's colour slightly changed [107].

Recently, researchers are involved in finding out new alternatives to control or reduce methane production in ruminants. Methane is considered a potent greenhouse gas because that represents a huge impact on the global warming effect (~25 times more potent than CO_2) [108]. Cinnamon leaf [109] and bark oils [110] has been tested in *in vitro* conditions to reduce the methane production. Both studies attributed an inhibition in the methanogenesis without adversely affecting the production of volatile fatty acids at different concentrations of cinnamon oils. Those studies reported that eugenol [109] and cinnamaldehyde [110] were the main metabolites causing a direct effect on methanogenesis.

Cinnamon oils could be used in mixtures with other components, even other oils obtained for spices. That approach was used to explore alternatives against *Rhipicephalus microplus* under *in vitro* tests using mixtures composed by cinnamon (*C. zeylanicum*). Thus, interesting findings have been reported with the following mixture cinnamon: all spices of, *i.e.* the cinnamaldehyde contributed to 37.7% of the total compounds in the mixture and the combination showed the highest acaricidal effect against *R. micropolus* [111].

Few studies investigated different presentations of cinnamon in the productive performance in the livestock. The cinnamon powder and essential oil were mixed with the feed of Japanese quails at doses of 1 and 2 g/kg and 100 and 200 mg/kg, respectively. The latter dose improves several parameters in quails such as feed conversion ratio, body weight gain, and antioxidant properties [112].

ADVANCES AND PERSPECTIVES OF CINNAMON IN THE CONTROL OF HELMINTHS

In general, the secondary metabolites responsible for the anthelmintic effect of plants can be classified into three main groups: terpenes (mono and sesquiterpenes, saponins and glycosides), phenolic compounds (tannins and flavonoids: anthocyanins, flavones, flavonols and isoflavonoids) and nitrogen-containing compounds (alkaloids and non-protein amino acids) [113 - 115]. Some compounds with antihelmintic activity isolated from plants are the steroidal saponins trillin and gracillin from *Dioscorea zingiberensis* [116 - 119]; the flavonoids sutchuenoside A and kaempferitrin from *Dryopteris crassirhizoma* [120]; and the triterpene saikosaponin. A from *Radix bupleuri* [121]. However, due to their toxicity, these compounds have limited potential for therapeutic use.

The use of these natural mixtures instead of synthetic drugs has many advantages; for example, the presence of several bioactive compounds that often act synergistically to achieve a therapeutic effect. Also, the use of whole extracts substantially reduces the risk of developing helminth resistance. Furthermore, plants and their derivatives are a good source of nutrients that bring additional benefits to the body that consumes them [115]. Therefore, steps have been taken towards the development of herbal remedies as a safer alternative to treat helminthiasis [113].

In this regard, a wide variety of aromatic plants belonging to the genus *Cinnamomum* offer the opportunity to study whole extracts and bioactive compounds to develop safe and effective alternative treatments for helminth parasitosis.

PERSPECTIVES ON THE STUDY OF THE ANTHELMINTIC PROPERTIES OF CINNAMON

Due to the nature of its chemical composition, cinnamon and its varieties have multiple medicinal properties. These properties are focused mainly on human health; however, this spice also has great potential to be used in animal and plant health. The research work reported to date indicates that *Cinnamomum verum* and other species of the genus have the potential to be used in the treatment of parasitic diseases caused by helminths. However, in order to transcend the knowledge of what has been done so far, there are aspects that need to be addressed.

Different studies have demonstrated the *in vitro* efficacy of plant extracts and essential oils against helminths. These products could be a source of new substances for the development of effective options for the treatment of helminthiasis. However, few studies have determined the identity of the chemical component, causing the activity. Chemical identification of bioactive compounds is essential to achieve reproducible formulations with continued efficacy. Furthermore, the identification of bioactive molecules can be useful for their application as lead compounds in the development of deworming drugs. The use of nuclear magnetic resonance spectroscopy and mass spectrometry will make a decisive contribution in this respect.

Most of the extracts and compounds are evaluated against parasitic nematodes in *in vitro* tests, but very few are examined by *in vivo* models, so the feasibility of their actual application is not known. As reported by Liu [122] in their review, of the 34 anthelmintic compounds reported so far, only eight have been evaluated *in vivo* models. *In vivo* evaluations are indispensable to propose the clinical development of the evaluated compounds. Also, the results of these evaluations are useful to validate the bioactivity of a plant that is used empirically. In this aspect, it is necessary to highlight the need to choose the most appropriate *in vivo* model and to carry out the trials in a controlled manner.

Likewise, to make the practical use of plant extracts, essential oils or bioactive compounds of cinnamon possible, it is necessary to investigate their systemic action in the host organism, determine their toxicity and study their mechanism of action. In this last aspect, the free-living nematode *Caenorhabditis elegans* can be used as a model organism.

On the other hand, most studies on the antiparasitic properties of cinnamon focus on studying the effect of its volatile phenolic compounds. However, as has been shown from the phytochemical analysis of the spice, cinnamon has plant compounds from other chemical classes that could have nematicidal activity, so this could be a fertile area for future research.

Finally, in the study of biologically active plants, it is interesting to explore possible synergistic and additive effects. The combined application of extracts and essential oils of cinnamon with those of another plant of known activity, even with the drugs used to treat parasitosis, could offer interesting and useful results in practice.

CONCLUSIONS

In this chapter, relevant information on various topics such as biology of cinnamon, traditional and molecular taxonomic description of cinnamon, metabolites present in cinnamon, uses of cinnamon as a condiment, antiparasitic properties of cinnamon, anthelmintic properties against agricultural pests, anthelmintic properties against livestock pests and productive performance, advances and perspectives of cinnamon in the control of anthelmintic properties, and perspectives on the study of the anthelmintic properties of cinnamon is presented. Further study of the antiparasitic properties of *Cinnamonum* extracts is required. Since its activity has been observed in some helminths, it can be a good alternative to the treatment of diseases caused by them. Because vaccines do not work in most cases and parasites sometimes become resistant to available synthetic therapies, it is important to seek alternative sources of parasitic disease medications.

Antiparasitic drugs that are effective and non-toxic to humans are often difficult to find, and on the other hands the plants produce a great diversity of products such as, secondary metabolites.

In this chapter, reports have been compiled on the efficacy of extracts of *Cinnamomum* spp. with antiprotozoal activity, mainly against *Plasmodium falciparum*, *Babesia* sp, *Theileria* and *Trypanosoma cruzi*; these extracts interfere with central targets of the parasites that results in the inhibition of the growth of some stages of the infection. Also, there are extracts with activity against helminths; that is why research on the efficacy of these extracts should be continued.

Therefore, several researchers advocate expanding, rather than decreasing, nature exploration as a source of new active agents that can serve as guides and platforms for the development of effective drugs needed for many diseases.

CONSENT FOR PUBLICATION

Not applicable.

CONFLICT OF INTEREST

The authors confirm that the contents of this chapter have no conflict of interest.

ACKNOWLEDGEMENTS

The present review article was partially financed by the National Problems project, Consejo Nacional de Ciencia y Tecnología, México (CONACYT) project number 9342634372.

REFERENCES

[1]   Mahmud R, Lim YAL, Amir A. Protozoa and helminths. Medical Parasitology. Cham: Springer 2018.

[2]   Hotez PJ, Brindley PJ, Bethony JM, King CH, Pearce EJ, Jacobson J. Helminth infections: the great neglected tropical diseases. J Clin Invest 2008; 118(4): 1311-21.
[http://dx.doi.org/10.1172/JCI34261] [PMID: 18382743]

[3]   Dante S, Zarlenga S, Hober EP, Detwiler JT. Diversity and history as drivers of helminth systematics and biology. In: Bruschi Fabrizio, Ed. Helminth Infections and their Impact on Global Public Health. Dipartimento di Ricerca Traslazionale, N.T.M.C. Universita`di Pisa. Pisa, Italy: Springer 2014; pp. 1-28.

[4]   Freeman MC, Akogun O, Belizario V Jr, *et al.* Challenges and opportunities for control and elimination of soil-transmitted helminth infection beyond 2020. PLoS Negl Trop Dis 2019; 13(4): e0007201.
[http://dx.doi.org/10.1371/journal.pntd.0007201] [PMID: 30973872]

[5]   Arsenopoulos K, Minoudi S, Symeonidou I, *et al.* Frequency of resistance to benzimidazoles of *Haemonchus contortus* helminths from dairy sheep, goats, cattle and buffaloes in Greece. Pathogens 2020; 9(5): 347.
[http://dx.doi.org/10.3390/pathogens9050347] [PMID: 32375252]

[6]   Finimundy TC, Pereira C, Dias MI, *et al.* Infusions of herbal blends as promising sources of phenolic compounds and bioactive properties. Molecules 2020; 25(9): 2151.
[http://dx.doi.org/10.3390/molecules25092151] [PMID: 32375427]

[7]   Domínguez F. La biotecnología y las plantas medicinales. México: Ciencia. CDMX 2015; p. 83.

[8]   Batiha GES, Beshbishy AM, Guswanto A, *et al.* Phytochemical characterization and chemotherapeutic potential of *Cinnamomum verum* extracts on the multiplication of protozoan parasites *in vitro* and *in vivo*. Molecules 2020; 25(4): 996.
[http://dx.doi.org/10.3390/molecules25040996] [PMID: 32102270]

[9]   Barceloux DG. Medical Toxicology of Natural Substances: Foods, Fungi, Medicinal Herbs, Toxic Plants, and Venomous Animals. Hoboken, NJ: John Wiley & Sons 2008; pp. 39-43.
[http://dx.doi.org/10.1002/9780470330319.ch4]

[10]   Wijesekera ROB. The chemistry and technology of cinnamon. CRC Crit Rev Food Sci Nutr 1978; 10: 1-30.
[http://dx.doi.org/10.1080/10408397809527243] [PMID: 363362]

[11]   Silva KTD, Ed. A manual on the essential oil Industry. Vienna, Austria: UNIDO 1995.

[12]   Maistre J. Las Plantas De Especias. Segunda ed. Barcelona: Editorial Blume 2000.

[13]   Souto da Rosa R, Numata R, Marovic ME, *et al.* Análisis Micrográfico y Fitoquímico De muestras Comerciales De "Canela". Dominguezla 2014; 31: 11-5.

[14]   Claus EP, Tyler VE. (h). *Farmacognosia.* 5ª edición. El Ateneo, Buenos Aires: 1968; 179-80.

[15]   Pillai NB. Export of spice oils from India - problems and prospects. Indian Perfumer 1993; 37(1): 94-110.

[16]   Bavappa KVA, Ruettimann RA. Cinnamon cultivation and processing. tech. bull.5. UNDP/FAO research project on minor export crops. dept. of minor export crops. Sri Lanka. 1981.

[17]   Radhakrishnan VV. Cinnamon - the spicy bark. Spice India 1992; 5(4): 11-3.

[18]   Thomas and Mathew. Cinnamon (*Cinnamomum verum* Presl.) for flavour and fragrance. KERALA

AGRICULTURAL UNIVERSITY, Aromatic & Medicinal Plants Research Station 2016.

[19] Krishnamoorthy B, Rema J, Zacharia TJ, Abraham J, Gopalam A. Navashree and nithyashree - two new high yielding and high-quality cinnamon (*Cinnamomum verum* Bercht & Presl.) Selections. J Spices Aromat Crops 1996; 5(1): 28-33.

[20] Kueffer C, Schumacher E, Fleischmann K, Edwards PJ, Dietz D. Una fuerte competencia bajo tierra moldea la regeneración De Los árboles En Los Bosques Invasores De *Cinnamomum verum*. Rev Ecol 2007; 95(2): 273-82.
[http://dx.doi.org/10.1111/j.1365-2745.2007.01213.x]

[21] Shu-Miaw C, Yu-Ching L, Yu-Wei W, *et al*. Stout camphor ttree genome fills gaps in understanding of flowering plant genome evolution. Nat Plants 2019; 5(1): 63-73.
[http://dx.doi.org/10.1038/s41477-018-0337-0]

[22] Lodish H. Berk, Matsudaria, Kaiser, Krieger, Scoot, Zipursky, Darnell Biología celular y molecular Lodish. Buenos Aires: Médica Panamericana 2005.

[23] Doh EJ, Kim JH, Oh SE, Lee G. Identification and Monitoring of Korean Medicines Derived from *Cinnamomum* spp. by Using ITS and DNA Marker. Genes Genomics 2017; 39(1): 101-9.
[http://dx.doi.org/10.1007/s13258-016-0476-5] [PMID: 28090265]

[24] Thu NT, Phuong NT, Ngoc NV. Cinnamomum sp 2019. https://www.ncbi.nlm.nih.gov/nuccore/MN852288.1

[25] Kress WJ, Wurdack KJ, Zimmer EA, Weigt LA, Janzen DH. Use of DNA barcodes to identify flowering plants. Proc Natl Acad Sci USA 2005; 102(23): 8369-74.
[http://dx.doi.org/10.1073/pnas.0503123102] [PMID: 15928076]

[26] Kress WJ, Erickson DL. A two-locus global dna barcode for land plants: the coding *rbcL* gene complements the non-coding *trnH-psbA* spacer region. PLoS One 2007; 2(6): e508.
[http://dx.doi.org/10.1371/journal.pone.0000508] [PMID: 17551588]

[27] Senanayake UM, Lee TH, Wills RBH. Volatile constituents of cinnamon (*Cinnamomum zeylanicum*) oils. J Agric Food Chem 1978; 26(4): 822-4.
[http://dx.doi.org/10.1021/jf60218a031]

[28] Jirovetz L, Buchbauer G, Ruzicka J, Shafi MP, Rosamma MK. Analysis of *Cinnamomum zeylanicum* blume leaf oil from South India. J Essent Oil Res 2001; 13(6): 442-3.
[http://dx.doi.org/10.1080/10412905.2001.9699721]

[29] Wang R, Wang R, Yang B. Extraction of essential oils from five cinnamon leaves and identi fication of their volatile compound compositions. Innov Food Sci Emerg Technol 2009; 10(2): 289-92.
[http://dx.doi.org/10.1016/j.ifset.2008.12.002]

[30] Isogai A, Suzuki A, Tamura S, Murakoshi S, Ohashi Y, Sasada Y. Structures of cinnzeylanine and cinnzeylanol, polyhydroxylated pentacyclic diterpenes from *cinnamomum zeylanicum* Nees. Agric Biol Chem 1976; 40(11): 2305-6.

[31] Jayaprakasha GK, Jagan Mohan Rao L, Sakariah KK, Akariah KUKS. Volatile constituents from *Cinnamomum zeylanicum* fruit stalks and their antioxidant activities. J Agric Food Chem 2003; 51(15): 4344-8.
[http://dx.doi.org/10.1021/jf034169i] [PMID: 12848508]

[32] Jayaprakasha GK, Rao LJ, Sakariah KK. Chemical composition of the volatile oil from the fruits of *Cinnamomum zeylanicum* blume. Flavour Fragrance J 1997; 12: 331-3.
[http://dx.doi.org/10.1002/(SICI)1099-1026(199709/10)12:5<331::AID-FFJ663>3.0.CO;2-X]

[33] Khuwijitjaru P, Sayputikasikorn N, Samuhasaneetoo S, Penroj P, Siriwongwilaichat P, Adachi S. Subcritical Water Extraction of Flavoring and Phenolic Compounds from Cinnamon bark (*cinnamomum zeylanicum*). J Oleo Sci 2012; 61(6): 349-55.
[http://dx.doi.org/10.5650/jos.61.349] [PMID: 22687781]

[34]   Jayaprakasha GK, Ohnishi-Kameyama M, Ono H, Yoshida M, Jaganmohan Rao L. Phenolic constituents in the fruits of *Cinnamomum zeylanicum* and their antioxidant activity. J Agric Food Chem 2006; 54(5): 1672-9.
[http://dx.doi.org/10.1021/jf052736r] [PMID: 16506818]

[35]   Wu T, Leu Y-L, Chan Y-Y, Yu S-M, Teng C-M, Su J-D. Lignans and an aromatic acid from *Cinnamomum philippinense*. Phytochemistry 1994; 36(3): 785-8.
[http://dx.doi.org/10.1016/S0031-9422(00)89818-0]

[36]   Anderson RA, Broadhurst CL, Polansky MM, *et al*. Isolation and characterization of polyphenol type-a polymers from cinnamon with insulin-like biological activity. J Agric Food Chem 2004; 52(1): 65-70.
[http://dx.doi.org/10.1021/jf034916b] [PMID: 14709014]

[37]   Peng X, Cheng KW, Ma J, *et al*. Cinnamon bark proanthocyanidins as reactive carbonyl scavengers to prevent the formation of advanced glycation endproducts. J Agric Food Chem 2008; 56(6): 1907-11.
[http://dx.doi.org/10.1021/jf073065v] [PMID: 18284204]

[38]   Sun P, Wang T, Chen L, *et al*. Trimer procyanidin oligomers contribute to the protective effects of cinnamon extracts on pancreatic β-cells *In vitro*. Acta Pharmacol Sin 2016; 37(8): 1083-90.
[http://dx.doi.org/10.1038/aps.2016.29] [PMID: 27238208]

[39]   Li HT, Li WJ, Wu HM, Chen CY. Alkaloids from *Cinnamomum philippinense*. Nat Prod Commun 2012; 7(12): 1581-2.
[http://dx.doi.org/10.1177/1934578X1200701209] [PMID: 23413556]

[40]   Kao C, Cho C, Wu H, *et al*. Cinnapine, a new pyridine alkaloid from *Cinnamomum philippinense*. Chem Nat Compd 2015; 51(4): 633-4.
[http://dx.doi.org/10.1007/s10600-015-1396-3]

[41]   Masnon FF, Hassan NPS, Ahmad F. Aporphine alkaloids of *Cinnamomum mollissimum* and their bioactivities. Nat Prod Commun 2014; 9(1): 31-2.
[http://dx.doi.org/10.1177/1934578X1400900110] [PMID: 24660455]

[42]   Gellert E, Summons RE. Alkaloids of the genus *Cinnamomum*. Aust J Chem 1970; 23(10): 2095-9.
[http://dx.doi.org/10.1071/CH9702095]

[43]   CODEX. 2020. http://www.fao.org/fao-who-codexalimentarius/home/en/

[44]   García-Casal MN, Peña-Rosas JP, Malavé HG. Sauces, spices, and condiments: definitions, potential benefits, consumption patterns, and global markets. Ann N Y Acad Sci 2016; 1379(1): 3-16.
[http://dx.doi.org/10.1111/nyas.13045] [PMID: 27153401]

[45]   Vangalapati N, Sree Satya D. Surya Prakash, Avanigadda S. "A review on pharmacological activities and clinical effects of cinnamon species. Res J Pharm Biol Chem Sci 2012; 3(1): 653-63.

[46]   Subasinghe S, Hettiarachchi CS, Iddagoda N. *In vitro* Propagation of cinnamon (*Cinnamomum verum* Presl) using Embryos and *In vitro* axillary bud. JOAAT 2016; 3(3): 164-9.
[http://dx.doi.org/10.18178/joaat.3.3.164-169]

[47]   Rawat I, Verma N, Joshi K. Cinnamon *(Cinnamomum zeylanicum)*. medicinal plants in India: importance and cultivation. 2020; pp. 165-177 165-77.

[48]   Torres JET, Gassara F, Kouassi AP, Brar SK, Belkacemi K. Spice use in food: properties and benefits. Crit Rev Food Sci Nutr 2017; 57(6): 1078-88.
[http://dx.doi.org/10.1080/10408398.2013.858235]

[49]   Maheshwari RK, Chauhan AK, Gupta A, Sharma S. Cinnamon: an imperative spice for human confort. International Journal of Pharmaceutical Research and Bio-science 2013; 2(5): 131-45.

[50]   Rao PV, Gan SH. Cinnamon: a multifaceted medicinal plant. Evid Based Complement Alternat Med 2014; 2014: 642942.
[http://dx.doi.org/10.1155/2014/642942] [PMID: 24817901]

[51] Wink M. Medicinal plants: a source of anti-parasitic secondary metabolites. Molecules 2012; 17(11): 12771-91.
[http://dx.doi.org/10.3390/molecules171112771] [PMID: 23114614]

[52] Costa Júnior DB, Araújo JSC, de Mattos Oliveira L, *et al.* Identification of novel antiplasmodial compound by hierarquical virtual screening and *In vitro* assays. J Biomol Struct Dyn 2020; 1102(May): 1-9.
[http://dx.doi.org/10.1080/07391102.2020.1763837] [PMID: 32364060]

[53] Parvazi S, Sadeghi S, Azadi M, *et al.* The effect of aqueous extract of cinnamon on the metabolome of *Plasmodium falciparum* using 1HNMR spectroscopy. J Trop Med 2016; 2016: 3174841.
[http://dx.doi.org/10.1155/2016/3174841] [PMID: 26904134]

[54] Azeredo CMO, Santos TG, Maia BHL de NS, Soares MJ. *In vitro* biological evaluation of eight different essential oils against *Trypanosoma cruzi*, with emphasis on *Cinnamomum verum* essential oil. BMC Complement Altern Med 2014; 14(1): 309.
[http://dx.doi.org/10.1186/1472-6882-14-309] [PMID: 25148924]

[55] Ranasinghe P, Jayawardena R, Pigera S, *et al.* Evaluation of pharmacodynamic properties and safety of cinnamomum zeylanicum (*Ceylon cinnamon*) in healthy adults: a phase I clinical trial. BMC Complement Altern Med 2017; 17(1): 550.
[http://dx.doi.org/10.1186/s12906-017-2067-7] [PMID: 29282046]

[56] de Jong RM, Tebeje SK, Meerstein-Kessel L, *et al.* Immunity against sexual stage *Plasmodium falciparum* and *Plasmodium vivax* parasites. Immunol Rev 2020; 293(1): 190-215.
[http://dx.doi.org/10.1111/imr.12828] [PMID: 31840844]

[57] Wilson DW, Langer C, Goodman CD, McFadden GI, Beeson JG. Defining the timing of action of antimalarial drugs against *Plasmodium falciparum*. Antimicrob Agents Chemother 2013; 57(3): 1455-67.
[http://dx.doi.org/10.1128/AAC.01881-12] [PMID: 23318799]

[58] Narayanan A, Sindhe R. Drug resistance in *Plasmodium* sp. and novel antimalarial natural products-emerging trends. phytochemistry: An *in-silico* and *in-vitro*. Update 2019; 95-108.
[http://dx.doi.org/10.1007/978-981-13-6920-9_6]

[59] Nkanwen ERS, Ducret Awouafack M, Kezetas Bankeu JJ, Kamdem Wabo H, Alkarim Mustafa SA, Shaiq Ali M, *et al.* Constituents from the Stem Bark of *Cinnamomum zeylanicum* Welw. (Lauraceae) and their Inhibitory Activity Toward *Plasmodium falciparum* enoyl-ACP Reductase Enzyme. Rec Nat Prod 2013; 7(4): 296-301.

[60] Beshbishy AM, Batiha GES, Yokoyama N, Igarashi I. Ellagic acid microspheres restrict the growth of babesia and theileria *In vitro* and *Babesia microti In vivo*. Parasit Vectors 2019; 12(1): 269.
[http://dx.doi.org/10.1186/s13071-019-3520-x] [PMID: 31138282]

[61] Piacenza L, Peluffo G, Alvarez MN, Martínez A, Radi R. *Trypanosoma cruzi* antioxidant enzymes as virulence factors in chagas disease. Antioxid Redox Signal 2013; 19(7): 723-34.
[http://dx.doi.org/10.1089/ars.2012.4618] [PMID: 22458250]

[62] Yang F, Long E, Wen J, *et al.* Linalool, Derived from *Cinnamomum camphora* (L.) presl leaf extracts, possesses molluscicidal activity against *Oncomelania hupensis* and inhibits infection of *Schistosoma japonicum*. Parasit Vectors 2014; 7: 407.
[http://dx.doi.org/10.1186/1756-3305-7-407] [PMID: 25174934]

[63] Kim JI, Jeong YL, Lee S. Insecticidal activity of cinnamon essential oils, constituents, and (E)-cinnamaldehyde analogues against *Metcalfa pruinosa* Say (Hemiptera: Flatidae) nymphs and Adults. Korean J Appl Entomol 2015; 54(4): 375-82.
[http://dx.doi.org/10.5656/KSAE.2015.10.0.056]

[64] Haddi KL, Faroni RA, Olivera EE. Cinnamon oil. In: Nollet L, Rathove HS, Eds. Green pesticides handbook Essential oils for pest control. CRC Press 2017; pp. 151-84.

[http://dx.doi.org/10.1201/9781315153131-7]

[65] Jain PL. Acetylcholinesterase activity of *Cinnamon zeylanicum* extract. J Adv Pharm Educ Res 2017; 7(4): 482-5.

[66] Ribeiro-Santos RM, Andrade D, Madella AP, *et al.* Revisting an ancient spice with medicinal purposes: cinnamon. Trends Food Sci Technol 2017; 62: 154-69.
[http://dx.doi.org/10.1016/j.tifs.2017.02.011]

[67] Enan E. Insecticidal activity of essential oils: octopaminergic sites of action. Comp Biochem Physiol C Toxicol Pharmacol 2001; 130(3): 325-37.
[http://dx.doi.org/10.1016/S1532-0456(01)00255-1] [PMID: 11701389]

[68] Rattan RS. Mechanism of action of insecticidal secondary metabolites of plant origin. Crop Prot 2010; 29: 913-9210.
[http://dx.doi.org/10.1016/j.cropro.2010.05.008]

[69] Tong F, Coats JR. Quantitative structure-activity relationships of monoterpenoid binding activities to the housefly GABA receptor. Pest Manag Sci 2012; 68(8): 1122-9.
[http://dx.doi.org/10.1002/ps.3280] [PMID: 22461383]

[70] Gershenzon J, Croteau R. Terpenoids. In: Rosenthal GA, Berenbaum MR, Eds. Hervibores their interaction with secondary plant metabolites The Chemical participants. New York: Academic Press 1991; Vol. 1: pp. 165-219.
[http://dx.doi.org/10.1016/B978-0-12-597183-6.50010-3]

[71] Islam R, Khan RI, Al-Reza SM, Jeong YT, Song CH, Khalequzzaman M. Chemical composition and insecticidal properties of *Cinnamum aromaticum* (Nees) essential oil against the stored product beetle *Callosobruchus maculatus* (F.). J Sci Food Agric 2009; 89: 1241-6.
[http://dx.doi.org/10.1002/jsfa.3582]

[72] Jumbo LK, Haddi LRD, Faroni F, Heleno FG. Pinto, Olivera EE. Toxicity to, oviposition and population growth impairments of *Callosobruchus maculatus* exposed to clove and cinnamon essential oils. PLoS One 2018; 13(11): 1-15.
[http://dx.doi.org/10.1371/journal.pone.0207618]

[73] Haddi K, Oliveira EE, Faroni LR, Guedes DC, Miranda NN. Sublethal exposure to clove and cinnamon essential oils induces hormetic-like responses and disturbs behavioral and respiratory responses in *Sitophilus zeamais* (Coleoptera: Cuculionidae). J Econ Entomol 2015; 108(6): 2815-22.
[http://dx.doi.org/10.1093/jee/tov255] [PMID: 26318008]

[74] Ashouri SN, Shayesteh M, Maroufpoor A, Ebadollahi S. Ghasemzadeh. Toxicity and progeny reduction of potency of two powders spices, tumeric and Cinnamon on Adults of *Rhyzopertha dominica* (F.) and *Sitophilus granarius* (L.). Mun Ent Zool 2010; 5: 1096-103.

[75] Plata-Rueda A, Campos JM, da Silva Rolim G, *et al.* Terpenoid constituents of cinnamon and clove essential oils cause toxic effects and behavior repellency response on granary weevil, sitophilus granarius. Ecotoxicol Environ Saf 2018; 156: 263-70.
[http://dx.doi.org/10.1016/j.ecoenv.2018.03.033] [PMID: 29554611]

[76] Kim S, Roh J, Kim D, Lee H, Ahn Y. Insecticidal activities of aromatic plant extrtacts and essential oils against *Sitophilus oryzae* and *Callosobruchus chinensis*. J Stored Prod Res 2003; 39: 293-303.
[http://dx.doi.org/10.1016/S0022-474X(02)00017-6]

[77] Lee EJ, Kim JR, Choi DR, Ahn YJ. Toxicity of cassia and cinnamon oil compounds and cinnamaldehyde-related Compounds to *Sitophilus oryzae* (Coleoptera: Curculionidae). J Econ Entomol 2008; 101(6): 1960-6.
[http://dx.doi.org/10.1603/0022-0493-101.6.1960] [PMID: 19133480]

[78] Ali F, Khan J, Zada A, *et al.* Bio-insecticidal efficacy of botanical extracts of citronella and cinnamon against *Tribulium castaneum, Sitophilus oryzae* and *Drosophila melanogaster* Under Laboratory Conditions. Fresenius Environ Bull 2019; 28(4A): 3104-9.

[79] Li L, Lingyan G, Ting X, Xihong L. Insecticidal effects of the insecticide based on porous starch and cinnamon oil against *Sitophilus zeamais*. Adv Mat Res 2011; (160-162): 579-84.
[http://dx.doi.org/10.4028/www.scientific.net/AMR.160-162.579]

[80] Brari J, Thakur DR. Insecticidal efficacy of essential oil from *Cinnamomum zeylanicum* Blume and its two major constituens against *Callosobruchus maculatus* (F.) and *Sitophilus* oryzae (L.). J Agricul Technol 2015; 11(6): 1323-36.

[81] Jumbo LL, Faroni RD, Olivera EE, Pimentel MA, Silva GN. Potential use of clove and cinnamon essential oils to control the Bean Weevil, *Acanthoscelides obtectus* say, in small storage units. Ind Crops Prod 2014; 56: 27-34.
[http://dx.doi.org/10.1016/j.indcrop.2014.02.038]

[82] Jo HJ, Park KM, Min SC, Na JH, Park KH, Han J. Development of an anti-insect sachet using a polyvinyl alcohol-cinnamon oil polymer strip against *Plodia interpunctella*. J Food Sci 2013; 78(11): E1713-20.
[http://dx.doi.org/10.1111/1750-3841.12268] [PMID: 24245888]

[83] Park B, Lee M, Lee S, *et al.* Insecticidal activity of coriander and cinnamon oils prepared by various methods against three species of agricultural pests (*Myzus persicae, Tetranychus urticae* and *Plutella xylostella*). J Appl Biol 2017; 60(2): 137-40.
[http://dx.doi.org/10.3839/jabc.2017.023]

[84] Park IK, Lee HS, Lee SG, Park JD, Ahn YJ. Insecticidal and fumigant activities of cinnamomum cassia bark-derived materials against *Mechoris ursulus* (Coleoptera: attelabidae). J Agric Food Chem 2000; 48(6): 2528-31.
[http://dx.doi.org/10.1021/jf9904160] [PMID: 10888580]

[85] Ahmad FB, Mackeen MM, Ali A, Mashirun S, Yaacob M. Repellency of essential oils against the domiciliary cockroach, periplaneta Americana. Insect Sci Appl 1995; 6(3/4): 391-3.

[86] Phillips AK, Appel AG, Sims SR. Topical toxicity of essential oils to the German cockroach (Dictyoptera: Blattellidae). J Econ Entomol 2010; 103(2): 448-59.
[http://dx.doi.org/10.1603/EC09192] [PMID: 20429462]

[87] Sinthusiri J, Soonwera M. Efficacy of herbal essential oils as insecticides against the housefly, *Musca domestica* L. Southeast Asian J Trop Med Public Health 2013; 44(2): 188-96.
[PMID: 23691628]

[88] Boito J, Da Silva A, dos Reis J, *et al.* Insecticidal and repellent effect of cinnamon oil on flies associated with livestock. Rev Mvz Cordoba 2018; 23(2): 6628-36.

[89] Khater HF, Ali AM, Abouelella GA, *et al.* Toxicity and growth inhibition potential of vetiver, cinnamon, and lavender essential oils and their blends against larvae of the sheep blowfly, *Lucilia sericata*. Int J Dermatol 2018; 57(4): 449-57.
[http://dx.doi.org/10.1111/ijd.13828] [PMID: 29417554]

[90] Kasim N, Ismail S, Masdar ND, Hamid F, Nawawi WJ. Extraction and potential of cinnamon essential oil towars repellency and insecticidal activity. International Journal of Scientific and Research Publications 2014; 4(7): 1-15.

[91] Huang C, Fu JT, Liu YK, Cheng DM, Zhang ZX. The insecticidal and repellent activity of soil containing cinnamon leaf debris against red importes fire ant workers. Sociobiology 2015; 62(1): 46-51.
[http://dx.doi.org/10.13102/SOCIOBIOLOGY.V62I1.46-51]

[92] Mutalib N, Azis TM, Mohamad S, *et al.* The repellent and lethal effects of black pepper (*Piper nigrum*), Chili Pepper (*Capsicum annum*) and Cinnamon (*Cinnamomum zeylanicum*) extracts towars the odours house ant (*Tapinoma sessile*). J Eng Appl Sci (Asian Res Publ Netw) 2017; 12(8): 2710-4.

[93] Benelli G, Pavela R, Giordani C, *et al.* Acute and sub-lethal toxicity of eight essential oils of comercial interest against the filariasis mosquito *Culex quinquefasciatus* and the housefly *Musca domestica*. Ind

Crops Prod 2018; 112: 668-90.
[http://dx.doi.org/10.1016/j.indcrop.2017.12.062]

[94] Cheng SS, Liu JY, Huang CG, Hsui YR, Chen WJ, Chang ST. Insecticidal activities of leaf essential oils from *Cinnamomum osmophloeum* against three mosquito species. Bioresour Technol 2009; 100(1): 457-64.
[http://dx.doi.org/10.1016/j.biortech.2008.02.030] [PMID: 18396039]

[95] Thomas A, Mazigo HD, Manjurano A, Morona D, Kweka EJ. Evaluation of active ingredients and larvicidal activity of clove and cinnamon essential oils against anopheles gambiae (sensu lato). Parasit Vectors 2017; 10(1): 411-8.
[http://dx.doi.org/10.1186/s13071-017-2355-6] [PMID: 28874207]

[96] Khater HF, Geden CJ. Efficacy and repellency of some essential oils and their blends against larval and adult house flies, *Musca domestica* L. (Diptera: Muscidae). J Vector Ecol 2019; 44(2): 256-63.
[http://dx.doi.org/10.1111/jvec.12357] [PMID: 31729802]

[97] Na YE, Kim SI, Bang HS, Kim BS, Ahn YJ. Fumigant toxicity of cassia and cinnamon oils and cinnamaldehyde and structurally related compounds to *Dermanyssus gallinae* (Acari: Dermanyssidae). Vet Parasitol 2011; 178(3-4): 324-9.
[http://dx.doi.org/10.1016/j.vetpar.2011.01.034] [PMID: 21324598]

[98] Khater HF, Ramadan MY, El-Madawy RS. Lousicidal, ovicidal and repellent efficacy of some essential oils against lice and flies infesting water buffaloes in Egypt. Vet Parasitol 2009; 164(2-4): 257-66.
[http://dx.doi.org/10.1016/j.vetpar.2009.06.011] [PMID: 19596520]

[99] Hoste H, Torres-Acosta JF, Sandoval-Castro CA, *et al.* Tannin containing legumes as a model for nutraceuticals against digestive parasites in livestock. Vet Parasitol 2015; 212(1-2): 5-17.
[http://dx.doi.org/10.1016/j.vetpar.2015.06.026]

[100] Ventura Cordero J, Sandoval-Castro CA, Gozález-Pech PG, Torres-Acosta JFT, Capetillo-Leal CM, Santos-Ricalde RH. Nutracéuticos: ¿Qué Son y Para qué Sirven? Bioagrociencias 2016; 9(2): 19-26.

[101] Katiki LM, Barbieri AME, Araujo RC, Veríssimo CJ, Louvandini H, Ferreira JFS. Synergistic interaction of ten essential oils against *Haemonchus contortusIn vitro*. Vet Parasitol 2017; 243: 47-51.
[http://dx.doi.org/10.1016/j.vetpar.2017.06.008] [PMID: 28807309]

[102] Williams AR, Ramsay A, Hansen TV, *et al.* Anthelmintic activity of trans-cinnamaldehyde and a- and b-type proanthocyanidins derived from cinnamon (*Cinnamomum verum*). Sci Rep 2015; 5: 14791.
[http://dx.doi.org/10.1038/srep14791] [PMID: 26420588]

[103] Lee SH, Lillehoj HS, Jang SI, Lee KW, Bravo D, Lillehoj EP. Effects of dietary supplementation with phytonutrients on vaccine-stimulated immunity against infection with *Eimeria tenella*. Vet Parasitol 2011; 181(2-4): 97-105.
[http://dx.doi.org/10.1016/j.vetpar.2011.05.003] [PMID: 21676547]

[104] Jyoti , Singh NK, Singh H, Mehta N, Rath SS. *In vitro* assessment of synergistic combinations of essential oils against *Rhipicephalus* (*Boophilus*) *microplus* (Acari: Ixodidae). Exp Parasitol 2019; 201(201): 42-8.
[http://dx.doi.org/10.1016/j.exppara.2019.04.007] [PMID: 31034814]

[105] Setiyoningrum F, Priadi G, Afiati F. Supplementation of ginger and cinnamon extract into goat milk kefir.AIP Conference Proceedings. 2019; 2175: p. (1)020069.
[http://dx.doi.org/10.1063/1.5134633]

[106] Hameed A. Widespread acquisition of antimicrobial resistance of *Klebseilla pneumoniae* isolated from raw milk and the effect of cinnamon oil on such isolates. Int Food Res J 2017; 24(2): 876-80.

[107] Hamid OIA, Abdelrahman NAM. Effect of adding cardamom, cinnamon and fenugreek to goat's milk curd on the quality of white cheese during storage. Int J Dairy Sci 2012; 7(2): 43-50.
[http://dx.doi.org/10.3923/ijds.2012.43.50]

[108] Benchaar C, Greathead H. Essential oils and opportunities to mitigate enteric methane emissions from ruminants. Anim Feed Sci Technol 2011; 166: 338-55.
[http://dx.doi.org/10.1016/j.anifeedsci.2011.04.024]

[109] Chaves AV, He ML, Yang WZ, Hristov AN, McAllister TA, Benchaar C. Effects of essential oils on proteolytic, deaminative and methanogenic activities of mixed ruminal bacteria. Can J Anim Sci 2008; 88: 117-22.
[http://dx.doi.org/10.4141/CJAS07061]

[110] Macheboeuf D, Morgavi DP, Papon Y, Mousset JL, Arturo-Schaan M. Dose–response effects of essential oils on *In vitro* fermentation activity of the rumen microbial population. Anim Feed Sci Technol 2008; 145: 335-50.
[http://dx.doi.org/10.1016/j.anifeedsci.2007.05.044]

[111] Lazcano Díaz E, Padilla Camberos E, Castillo Herrera GA, *et al.* Development of essential oil-based phyto-formulations to control the cattle tick *Rhipicephalus microplus* using a mixture design approach. Exp Parasitol 2019; 201: 26-33.
[http://dx.doi.org/10.1016/j.exppara.2019.04.008] [PMID: 31029699]

[112] Mehdipour Z, Afsharmanesh M, Sami M. Effects of dietary synbiotic and cinnamon (Cinnamomum verum) supplementation on growth performance and meat quality in Japanese quail. Livest Sci 2013; 154(1-3): 152-7.
[http://dx.doi.org/10.1016/j.livsci.2013.03.014]

[113] Gogoi B, Kakoti BB, Bora NS, Yadav P. *In vitro* antihelmintic activity of bark extract of *Cinnamomum bejolghota* (Buch. -Ham.) in Indian adult earthworm (*Pheretima posthuma*). Asian Pac J Trop Dis 2014; 4 (Suppl. 2): S924-7.
[http://dx.doi.org/10.1016/S2222-1808(14)60759-3]

[114] Gaikwad SA, Kale AA, Jadhav BG, Deshpande NR, Salvekar JP. Anthelmintic activity of *Cassia auriculata* L. extracts-*In vitro* Study. J Nat Prod Plant Resour 2011; 1(2): 62-6.

[115] Zajíčková M, Nguyen LT, Skálová L, Raisová Stuchlíková L, Matoušková P. Anthelmintics in the future: current trends in the discovery and development of new drugs against gastrointestinal nematodes. Drug Discov Today 2020; 25(2): 430-7.
[http://dx.doi.org/10.1016/j.drudis.2019.12.007] [PMID: 31883953]

[116] Mukherjee N, Mukherjee S, Saini P, Roy P, Babu SP. Phenolics and terpenoids; the promising new search for anthelmintics: a critical review. Mini Rev Med Chem 2016; 16(17): 1415-41.
[http://dx.doi.org/10.2174/1389557516666151120121036] [PMID: 26586122]

[117] Scott I, Pomroy WE, Kenyon PR, Smith G, Adlington B, Moss A. Lack of efficacy of monepantel against *Teladorsagia circumcincta* and *Trichostrongylus colubriformis*. Vet Parasitol 2013; 198(1-2): 166-71.
[http://dx.doi.org/10.1016/j.vetpar.2013.07.037] [PMID: 23953148]

[118] Fabbri J, Maggiore MA, Pensel PE, Denegri GM, Elissondo MC. *In vitro* Efficacy study of *Cinnamomum zeylanicum* essential oil and cinnamaldehyde against the larval stage of *Echinococcus granulosus*. Exp Parasitol 2020; 214: 107904.
[http://dx.doi.org/10.1016/j.exppara.2020.107904] [PMID: 32371061]

[119] Wang GX, Jiang DX, Li J, Han J, Liu YT, Liu XL. Anthelmintic activity of steroidal saponins from *Dioscorea zingiberensis* C. H. Wright Against *Dactylogyrus Intermedius* (Monogenea) in Goldfish (*Carassius* Auratus). Parasitol Res 2010; 107(6): 1365-71.
[http://dx.doi.org/10.1007/s00436-010-2010-z] [PMID: 20689967]

[120] Jiang B, Chi C, Fu YW, Zhang QZ, Wang GX. *In vivo* anthelmintic effect of flavonol rhamnosides from *Dryopteris crassirhizoma* Against *Dactylogyrus intermedius* in Goldfish (*Carassius auratus*). Parasitol Res 2013; 112(12): 4097-104.
[http://dx.doi.org/10.1007/s00436-013-3600-3] [PMID: 24013342]

[121] Zhu S, Ling F, Zhang Q, *et al.* Anthelmintic activity of saikosaponins a and d from *radix bupleuri* Against *Dactylogyrus* spp. Infecting Goldfish. Dis Aquat Organ 2014; 111(2): 177-82.
[http://dx.doi.org/10.3354/dao02789] [PMID: 25266906]

[122] Liu M, Panda SK, Luyten W. Plant-based natural products for the discovery and development of novel anthelmintics against nematodes. Biomolecules 2020; 10(3): E426.
[http://dx.doi.org/10.3390/biom10030426] [PMID: 32182910]

CHAPTER 2

Nutraceutical Attributes of *Tamarindus indica* L. - Devils' Tree with Sour Date

S. Aishwarya[1], Kounaina Khan[2], Anirudh Gururaj Patil[1], Pankaj Satapathy[1], Aishwarya T. Devi[3], M.G. Avinash[4], S.M. Veena[5], Shubha Gopal[4], M.N. Nagendra[3], K. Muthucheliyan[1], Shivaprasad Hudeda[2], Farhan Zameer[1,*] and Sunil S. More[1,*]

[1] *School of Basic and Applied Sciences, Department of Biological Sciences, Dayananda Sagar University, Shavige Malleshwara Hills, Kumaraswamy Layout, Bengaluru - 560 111, Karnataka, India*

[2] *Department of Dravyaguna, JSS Ayurvedic Medical College, Lalithadripura, Mysuru - 570 028, Karnataka, India*

[3] *Department of Biotechnology, Sri Jayachamarajendra College of Engineering, JSS Science and Technology University, JSS Research Foundation, SJCE Campus, Manasagangothri, Mysore - 570 006, Karnataka, India*

[4] *Department of Studies in Microbiology, University of Mysore, Manasagangotri, Mysore – 570 006, Karnataka, India*

[5] *Department of Biotechnology, Sapthagiri College of Engineering, Bangalore - 560 057, India*

Abstract: *Tamarindus indica* L. (Fabaceae) plant has a dominion for its usage in culinary additional to medicinal and nutritional value globally. It is used as a preservative and savory in Indian dishes from time immemorial. Traditional nutritional constituents and its significance with respect to leaf, flower, fruits and seeds have been reported in folklore and Ayurvedic practice. This chapter primarily focuses on the various bioactivities (anti-microbial, anti-oxidant, anti-inflammatory, anti-cancer, anti-dote, anti-diabetic) and their probable known mode of action in combating the disorder/disease. Further, the structure-activity relationship (SAR) studies were performed with lead phytobioactives to understand potential pathways. However, with the tamarind fruit and seeds, many controversial myths also exist. This comprehensive chapter depicts and contemplates the unexplored science of this Devils' tree with Sour date which is extensively used in nutritional, pharmaceutical with pharmacological attributes with clinical significance "Making Food as Medicine".

* **Corresponding Authors Sunil S. More and Farhan Zameer:** School of Basic and Applied Sciences, Department of Biological Sciences, Dayananda Sagar University, Shavige Malleshwara Hills, Kumaraswamy Layout, Bengaluru - 560 111, Karnataka, India; Tel: 0091 - 8073246552; E-mail: drsunil@dsu.edu.in & School of Basic and Applied Sciences, Department of Biological Sciences, Dayananda Sagar University, Shavige Malleshwara Hills, Kumaraswamy Layout, Bengaluru - 560 111, Karnataka, India; Tel: 0091 - 9844576378; E-mail: farhanzameeruom@gmail.com

Atta-ur-Rahman, M. Iqbal Choudhary & Sammer Yousuf (Eds.)

Keywords: Biologicals, Functional food, Imli, Phytochemistry, Processing, Therapeutics.

INTRODUCTION

Tamarindus indica L. is an indigenous evergreen commercialized tropical, medicinal plant that belongs to the family *Fabaceae* or *Leguminosae* and the genus *Tamarindus* [1]. *Tamarindus indica*, commonly known as tamarind originated in tropical Africa and now is found in subtropical regions, India, Sudan, Nigeria, Tanzania and Zambia. Tamarind is proved to be underutilized worldwide [2] but it is found to have effective potential that addresses health, nutritional, environmental and socioeconomic constraints [3]. Tamarind grows into an evergreen tree with a height of 20-30m tall and a width of 1-2 m. The leaves of the plant are compound arranged in an alternate fashion with 10-18 pairs of leaflets. Tamarind is used all over the world since it is a pan-tropical species [4]. Tamarind is mostly used in making of kitchen equipment and agricultural tools due to its hard-wood [1]. The most commercial use of tamarind is food production and in traditional medicine due to its pharmacological and pharmacodynamic properties. The fruit of the plant is a pod that is subcylindrical, curved and rusty-brown embedded in a sticky pulp which is edible in nature. It is found to be rich in polysaccharides that are potent molecules with anti-mutagenic, anti-inflammatory, anti-diabetic, anti-oxidant, anti-hepatotoxic, digestive and laxative properties [5, 6]. *Tamarindus indica* consists of proteins, carbohydrates that help in building the capacity of the muscles. It is also found to be rich in magnesium, calcium, potassium, phosphorous and minerals and contains fewer amounts of vitamin A and iron. The phytochemical constituent of tamarind consists of cardiac glycosides [7], phenolic compounds, arabinose, galactose, tartaric acid, mucilage, glucose, uronic acid [8] and mallic acid [9]. It also contains some essential fatty acids and elements such as cadmium, manganese, lead, zinc, copper, arsenic, iron, potassium and calcium [10]. Tamarind is used in beverages, ethnoveterinary applications, food, ethnomedicines and aesthetic uses. This chapter describes the drug review, vernacular names in different languages, the biological, pharmacological, clinical and nutraceutical studies of the plant. This chapter also describes the structure of the potent phytomolecules and the structure-activity relationship of these molecules with various biomarkers that cause stress, inflammation, disorders and diseases which would be further explored as therapeutic targets for drug design and discovery.

BIOLOGICAL/PHARMACOLOGICAL/NUTRACEUTICAL ACTIVITIES OF SPICES AND CULINARY HERBS

Disorder or a disease is caused due to any malfunctioning in the normal functioning of an organism symptomatic or asymptomatic leading to an abnormal state. The normal functioning of the human body is impudent to understand so that any changes in this normal functioning could be analyzed to treat the disease [12]. Indian folklore literature gives us an insight that tamarind provides shade for livestock's, public places, homes and crops. Since it has a strong root system, it provides crops and houses a windbreak that is tamarind trees are never blown off by the wind and their branches never fall off. A number of superstitions, ownerships, taboos, beliefs and culture norms are associated with tamarind [1]. Only 3% of the tamarind tree belongs to public property and almost 85% of the tamarind is owned by men and only 12% by women. The ripened fruits are harvested by climbing and shaking the tree mostly by men or young children and the fruit fall are collected from the ground. The fruit pulp is soaked in water and softened to get a concentrate which is used in millet bread, potatoes and porridge. 'Tamarindade' is a drink that is enjoyed by small children by removing the seeds and adding the fruit to a bottle of water and shaking it. The seeds are roasted and used as a snack in the rural population where they give a similar taste as peanuts [32]. Since tamarind takes a long time to grow, it is believed that the children and the grandchildren can taste the tamarind rather the person who planted since they cannot live that long. Traditionally, the dead relatives are buried near the tamarind trees as an honor; therefore it brings a close relationship between the trees and culture. Girls who are in menstrual cycles and women are not allowed to climb tamarind trees since there was an experience where a girl climbed the tree when she was in the menstrual cycle and it was observed that the fruits became sour in Jopadhola ethnic group therefore it is believed as a taboo [12]. People avoid going near tamarind trees at night because it is believed that the spirit of the dead are vested in the tree and also sleeping in the shade of the tree is a prejudice since they give out unhealthy vapors. People need to recognize the actual uses of tamarind since it has a wide range of phytochemical composition that can treat a number of diseases. Prolonged use of chemical drugs is causing diverse range of side effects including decalcification in men and women after the age of 45 years. High amount of calcium is lost in women after menopause causing decalcification, osteoporosis, arthritis and fractures due to imbalance in estrogen the hormone for reproductive development. Ayurvedic systems of medicine do not give us the molecular mechanism of action of the phytomolecules therefore modern medicine needs to be understood to study the mechanism of the pharmacology and the pharmaceutical properties [1, 32]. The use of natural medicine for the treatment of diseases is a crucial need; therefore tamarind and its importance in treating diseases are enlisted in Table **1**.

METABOLIC DISORDERS

The process of breaking down of food into fats, proteins and carbohydrates to liberate energy is called metabolism. Metabolism takes place in the presence of enzymes and chemicals that degrade food particles into acids and sugars and use them as the body's fuel. Disorders or diseases are due to abnormal chemical reactions that take place during metabolism. Liver, pancreas and other organs get damaged due to metabolic disorders; lifestyle plays a major role in the development of metabolic disorders [13]. Major focus is required to find alternative natural medicine to treat diseases.

Table 1. Summary of bioactivity and vegetative components from *Tamarindus indica*.

Bioactivity	Plant Part Used	Organism	Reference
Anti-diabetic and Anti-oxidant activity	Seed coat	Rats	[16]
Anti-tuberculosis	Fruit	Wistar albino rats	[25]
Nephrotoxicity	Fruit	Male rabbits	[27]
Aphrodisiac activity	Pulp	Wistar rats	[35]
Hepatoprotective activity	Leaves	Sprague Dawley rats	[40, 41]
Snake bite	Seeds	Patients	[46]

Diabetes mellitus is a metabolic disorder that develops due to the lack of insulin production by the pancreatic cells [14]. Genetically engineered insulin is used to treat diabetes mellitus presently, but prolonged exposure is also found to cause severe side effects [15]. Ayurveda, the Indian traditional system of medicine, is used for the maintenance of diabetes [16]. In this study, the seeds of the tamarind were employed and the seed coats were separated and grinded, the obtained powder was soaked in ethanol. A hydroethanolic extract of the seed coat was prepared and subjected to phytochemical screening. The extract was found to contain glycosides, saponins, tannins, flavonoids and polyphenols. When 100 mg/kg of the extract was subjected to alloxan-induced hyperglycemic rats, the blood glucose level reduced significantly and also promoted the regeneration of β-cells in the pancreas [17]. Prolonged alloxan treatment is found to cause permanent damage to the β-cells or islet of Langerhans by inhibiting Ca^{2+} and calmodulin-dependent protein kinase decreasing the amount of insulin production [18]. From this study, it was concluded that the hydroethanolic extract of the seed coat had significant anti-diabetic properties and anti-oxidant activity [16].

TUBERCULOSIS

Tuberculosis (TB) is a very common bacterial disease worldwide caused by different strains of Mycobacterium tuberculosis [19]. Presently, the drugs used to treat tuberculosis include rifampicin (RIF), ethambutol, Isoniazid (INH), streptomycin and pyrazinamide (PZA) [20]. Hepatotoxicity or liver toxicity is doubled on treatment with isoniazid and rifampicin [21], leading to bilirubin leakage and other liver enzymes including alkaline phosphatase (ALP), serum glutamate oxaloacetate transaminase (SGOT) and serum glutamate pyruvate transaminase (SGPT) [22]. Therefore, it is crucial to develop new drugs that can ameliorate TB without causing any side effects [23]. Therefore, the use of naturally available phytomolecules from natural sources would be preferred since they would not cause any side effects. *Tamarindus indica* consists of biologically active molecules such as orientin, glycosides, hordenine and vitexin [24]. Aqueous extract of *Tamarindus indica* was tested against wistar albino rats that were induced with hepatotoxicity. When the aqueous extract was administered to the rats at a higher dosage, they exhibited significant hepatoprotective activity in individuals on anti-TB drugs. The probable mechanism could be the radical scavenging mechanism that provides hepatoprotection. Therefore, further studies need to be researched to identify the efficacy of the culinary herb and its therapeutic application [25].

NEPHROTOXICITY

Gentamycin is an antibacterial drug that is less prone to bacterial resistance [26] used against gram-negative bacteria. Though gentamycin has beneficial aspects, it is found to cause nephrotoxicity. According to the literature survey, the nephrotoxic effects of gentamycin can be ameliorated using tamarind. Tamarind consists of phenolic compounds and flavonoids that have potent anti-oxidant activity. The fruit of tamarind was employed for the study where the ethanolic extract of the fruit was administered to male rabbits. Rabbits induced with nephrotoxicity with the help of gentamycin were treated with the tamarind extract. The functional parameters of the kidney such as blood urea nitrogen, urinary volume, serum creatinine, body weight, urinary excretion of proteins and lactate dehydrogenase reduced significantly providing nephroprotective activity at a dosage of 200 mg/kg. Therefore, successful nephroprotective properties were observed in animals induced with gentamycin-nephrotoxic effects [27].

APHRODISIAC ACTIVITY

Reproductive disorders such as sexual dysfunction are a major public health concern that is causing social and serious medical problems affecting 25-63% of females and 10-52% of males [28]. The quality of sperm in males has a sharp decline in the last 50 years [29, 30]. The parameters associated to this decline include socioeconomic status, stress, nutrition, sedentary lifestyle and environment [31]. Diet plays a major role in the quality of sexual life; therefore, following a decorous nutritious diet is mandatory for proper health. In this study, tamarind was used due to the presence of high phenolic content that exhibits high anti-oxidant capacity [32, 33]. In Ayurveda, the kernel of tamarind along with ajwain, is used to enhance the sperm count and also to treat premature ejaculation [34]. Tamarind fruits were collected and an aqueous extract of the same was prepared and administered to wistar rats of either sex. Catechin, gallic acid was present in high amounts in the extract prepared and exhibited effective treatment for reproductive disorders when compared to the standard sildenafil citrate. Tamarind at a dosage of 125 mg/kg and 250 mg/kg increased the aphrodisiac potential in these rats and did not produce any toxic effects on the testis and sperm quality [35].

HEPATOPROTECTIVE ACTIVITY

High levels of reactive oxygen species (ROS) and reactive nitrogen species (RNS) lead to oxidative stress leading to damage of all the types of biomolecules such as proteins, enzymes, lipids, carbohydrates, DNA and amino acids [36]. In normal condition, there is a proper balance between antioxidants and oxidants, any kind of disturbance to this equilibrium leads to oxidative stress contributing to the pathogenesis of a number of diseases. The liver cells are damaged leading to hepatic damage by the production of ROS that overpowers the immune system through hepatotoxic chemicals [37]. Tamarind leaves are used to make a decoction that is used to treat gallbladder disorders, hepatitis and jaundice in the Amazon and the Caribbean parts [38]. Tamarind majorly constitutes antioxidant molecules; therefore for centuries, it has been used as a hepatoprotective agent. In a study, tamarind leaves were obtained and optimized into tablets by wet granulation method [39]. These tablets were administered to female Sprague Dawley rats and tested for its anti-oxidant and hepatoprotective activity. The anti-oxidant defense system is activated by these tablets, where elements like palmitic, tartaric, citric, lupeol, lupanone, malic acids, iron and manganese also contribute to the anti-oxidant ability [40, 41]. It reduced the cholesterol and the triglyceride levels and increased the HDL-c content in the rats. The tamarind tablets maintained the liver functioning at a concentration of 200 mg/kg proving that tamarind has hepatoprotection activity.

SNAKEBITE

Snakebite is causing a major death rate in the tropical countries and as well as in India it is the most basic cause of mortality due to high amount of fear and stress.

The statistical analysis estimates that in India 35,000 to 50,000 people are dying due to snakebite [42]. *Naja naja* (Cobra), *Daboia russelli* (Russell's viper), *Bangarus caeruleus* (Krait) and *Echis carinatus* (Saw-scaled viper) are the most common poisonous snakes that are found in India [43, 44]. Various plants having medicinal properties have been used in the treatment of snakebite, including tamarind [45]. The folklore literature explains a method of treatment for the snakebites. Tamarind seeds are crushed and soaked in alcohol, especially rum or brandy for about 30 minutes and the obtained product is filtered through a muslin cloth or a sieve. The obtained filtrate is diluted with water and the patient will be treated by giving 2 table-spoons orally, it is used at the site of the wound and tropical application, this method is used as a first aid to treat any venomous snake bite [46]. The powder of the plant was made and a spoonful of this powder was mixed with honey and taken orally three times a day every two hours to treat snakebite by the aboriginals of Jalgaon district [47]. Viper venom is one of the most poisonous venom in India that consists of toxic proteins including myotoxins, proteolytic enzymes, phospholipase A_2, cytotoxins and neurotoxins [48]. In India, medicinal plants that consist of pharmacologically active components have been used to treat snake envenomation [49]. Ethanol extract of the tamarind seeds was used to treat this venom where 7.5µg of the extract completely inhibited the hydrolytic enzymes particularly phospholipase A_2. The extract inhibited the enzyme through chelation of Ca^{2+} by direct binding. This study concludes that tamarind consists of potent phytomolecules that have the ability to neutralize snake envenomation [50].

PHYTOCHEMISTRY OF SPICES AND CULINARY HERBS

The enormously used phytomolecules present in *Tamrindus indica* including β-sitosterol, catechin, lupeol and naringenin are known for its therapeutic activities and can also be isolated from different plants (Fig. **1**). β-sitosterol and lupeol phytomolecules have been isolated, purified, and characterized by our lab for the first time from *Musa* sp. var. Nanjangud Rasa Bale [51]. These molecules were tested for their anti-diabetic activity in wistar rats induced with diabetes with the help of alloxan. Lupeol is a triterpenoid that was isolated from the inflorescence whereas β-sitosterol is a phytosterol that was isolated from the pseudostem of the plant. When these molecules were administered into diabetic rats they enhanced the production of insulin by restoring β-cells and also positively regulated glycogen storage pathways and glucose utilization. These molecules are not only found to have anti-diabetic properties but also anti-oxidant [52], anti-hyperglycemic [53]. Catechin is a flavonoid that is a major component of green tea that can be isolated from tea plant and barley [54], it is also used to treat cancer [55]. Naringenin is also a flavonoid that is present in citrus fruits; it is used to treat a number of diseases since it has high medicinal value. Naringenin induces apoptosis and regulates the mitogen activated protein kinase pathway by inhibiting growth factors like TGF-β (tumor growth factor- β) and VEGF (vascular endothelial growth factor) to protect from hepatocellular carcinoma [56]. It is also used to treat diabetes [57], breast cancer [58], dengue virus replication [59] and accumulation of diacylglycerol in skeletal muscles [60].

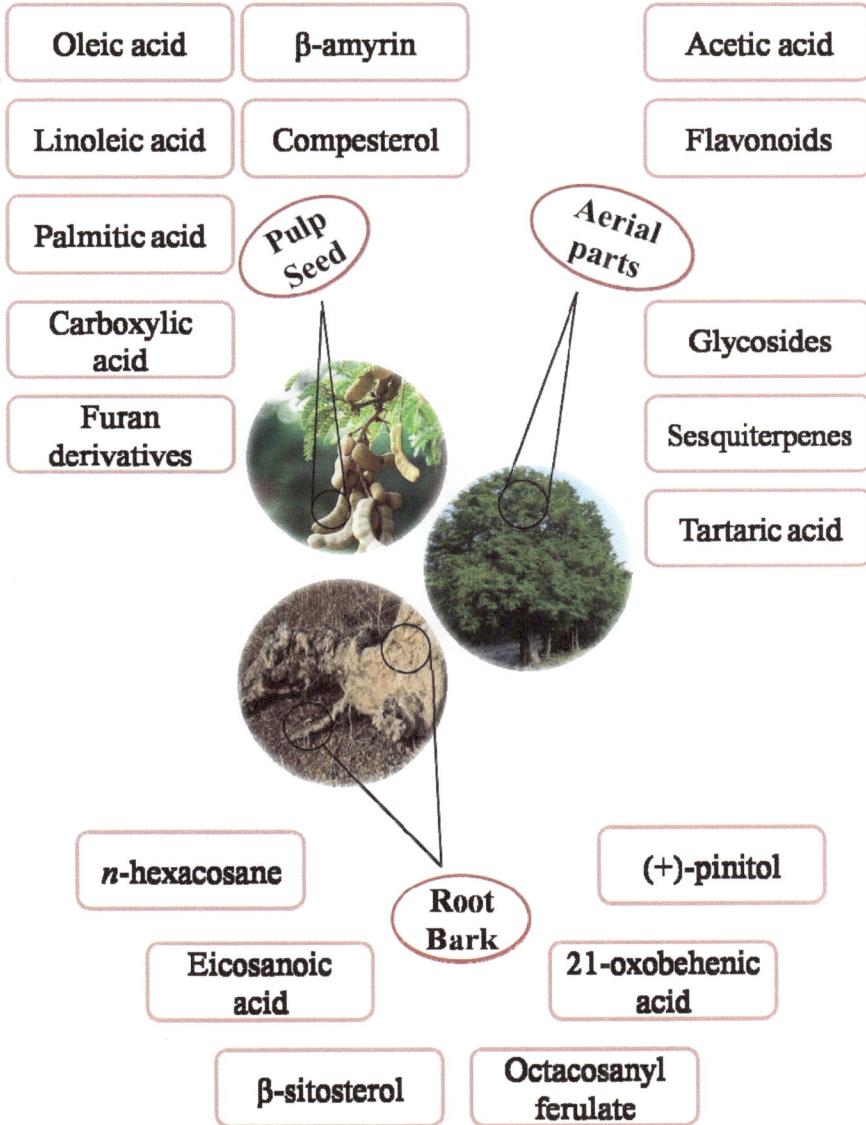

Fig. (1). Phytomolecules associated with Tamarind tree.

In all the studies that have been executed, *in silico* studies of the phytomolecules present in *Tamrindus indica* has not been performed, in order to provide a new criterion to the paper, structure and activity relationship studies has been performed. The top phytomolecules and their activity have been represented below correspondingly (Fig. **2**). These studies give an insight about the potent phytomolecules that is present in different parts of the plants and their bioactivities. The efficient targets of different disorders or diseases have been selected for the study. The result gives us a corollary to perform the wet lab experiments and to prove the results.

STRUCTURE-ACTIVITY RELATIONSHIP (SAR) STUDIES

Molecular docking studies were executed to establish a correlation between the top four potent phytomolecules (lupeol, β-sitosterol, catechin and naringenin) present in tamarind. Any disorder has three major common pathways including stress leading to inflammation and finally a disease. Therefore all the three pathways were chosen and the targets were screened and SAR studies were performed. Stress related targets superoxide dismutase was employed for the study with accession number in RCSB protein data bank (PDB): 2ADQ. Inflammatory targets such as cyclooxygenase-2 and lipooxygenase with accession number 1CX2 and 1YGE were chosen respectively. Diabetes targets aldol reductase and ACC2 with accession number 4JIR and 3JRW, ulcer and liver biomarkers such as sodium potassium ATPase and alkaline phophatase and aspartate amino transferase with accession number 1MO7 and 1EW2, 3WZF were preferred for the study respectively. The potent phytomolecules (ligands) were docked into the active site using Molecular docking software PATCH Dock with default parameters. PATCH Dock is an algorithm that is used to calculate the docking modes of small molecules into the active sites based on the shape complementarity. Molecular docking of the molecules revealed the atomic contact energy (ACE) and the amino acid binding residues that are as depicted in Tables below. The structures of the ligands were constructed using Dundee PRODRG server [61] which reduces the energy and standardizes the conformation of the side chains. The precise location of the binding site and the potentiality of the ligand to bind to the active site were determined using an automated docking software, molegro virtual docker 2008, version 3.2.1 (Molegro ApS, Aarhus, Denmark, http://molegro.com), that is based on guided differential evolution and a force filed based screening function [62]. With the help of Clustering methods the possible binding conformations and orientations were determined. The enzyme was visualized using the sequence option. The binding site was calculated within a spacing range so that the binding site was well sampled with a grid resolution of 0.3Å. Using MolDock optimizer algorithm the ligand was docked into the grid and the interactions were analyzed using detailed energy estimates. The software was utilized to identify hydrogen bonds and hydrophobic interactions between residues at the active site and the ligand.

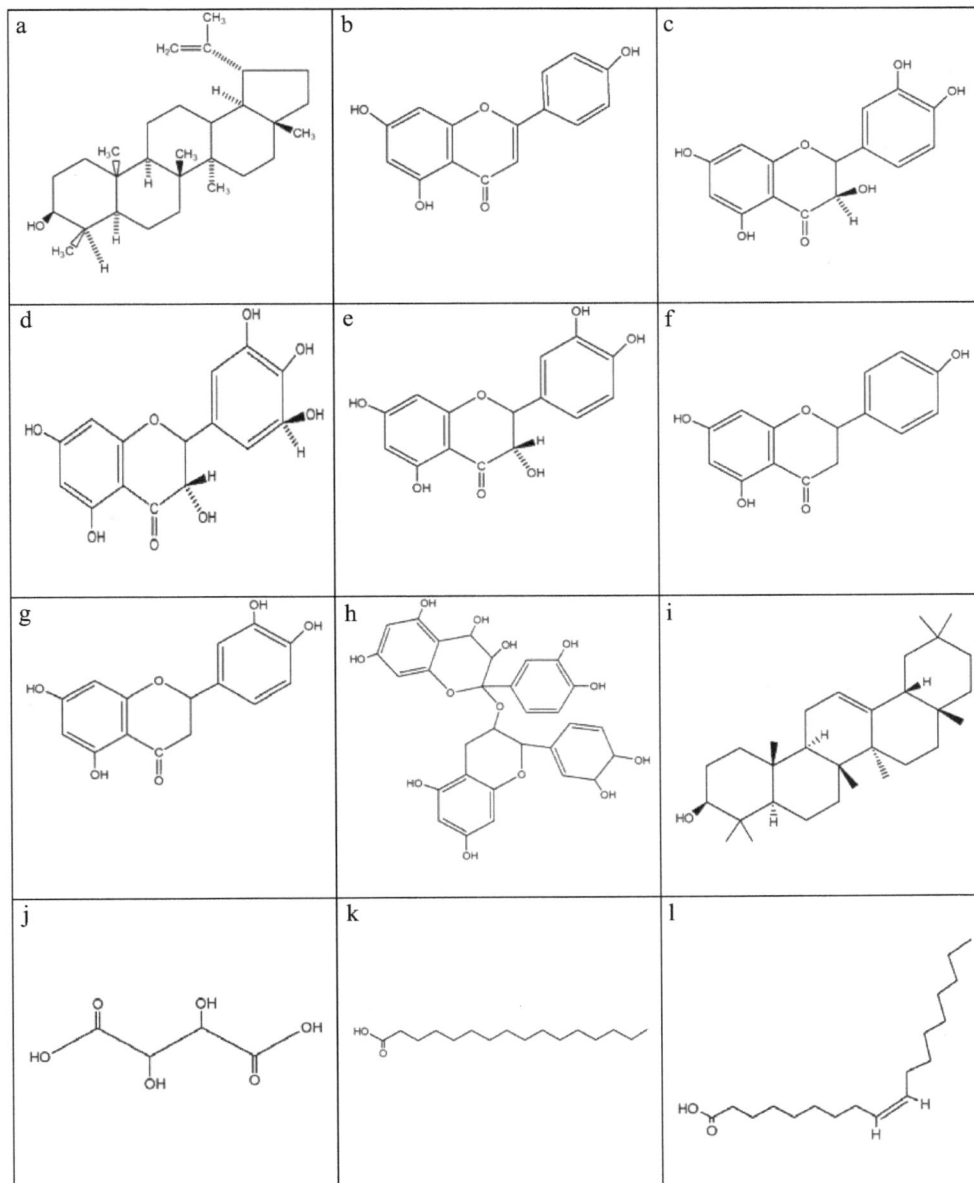

Fig. (2). (**a**) Lupeol, (**b**) apigenin, (**c**) catechin, (**d**) taxifolin, (**e**) epicatechin, (**f**) naringenin, (**g**) eriodictin, (**h**) procyanidin, (**i**) β-amyrin, (**j**) tartaric acid, (**k**) palmitic acid, (**l**) oleic acid.

MOLECULAR DOCKING STUDIES

Stress Biomarkers

The major biomarker of any disorder or disease is symptoms, the basic dysfunction that our body expresses. Once these symptoms are neglected it leads to stress that causes the release of excessive reactive oxygen species (ROS) that is responsible for any disorder or diseases. Superoxide dismutase (SOD) is the first line of defense against ROS that constitute one of the most important anti-oxidant molecules in the human body [63]. SOD can be a major biomarker that can be targeted to ameliorate oxidative stress that can lead to many other consequences. Fig. (**3**) depicts the SAR studies of SOD with lead phytobioactives and the results have been tabulated in Table **2**.

Table 2. Docking sites and there atomic contact energy values for stress disorder.

Name of the Biomarker	Name of the Compound	Details of H-bond Interaction	Atomic Contact Energy (ACE)	Amino Acid Residues on Docked Domains
		No. of Bond	Values	
SOD (superoxide dismutase) (2ADQ)	β-sitosterol	0	-337.59	Cys 44, Ser 46, Ile 183, Gly 251, Val 272, Gly 273, Leu 274, Val 296
	Catechin	12	-527.86	Cys 44, Gly 45, Ser 46, Ile 56, Gly 57, Asn 58, Phe 59, Ile 256, Leu 271, Gly 273, Leu 274, Thr 279, Val 296, Val 272, Ser 276, Arg 298, Phe 297
	Lupeol	0	-238.30	Cys 44, Ser 46, Ile 56, Phe 59, Val 159, Arg 298, Leu 274, Phe 297
	Naringenin	2	-212.65	Thr 202, Leu 204, Ala 254, Glu 226
	Donazepril	5	-365.13	Val 159, Gly 251, Val 272, Gly 272, Leu 274, Gly 275, Ser 276, Thr 279, Val 296, Phe 297, Arg 298

The results exhibited catechin had the highest ACE value of -527.86 among the top 4 phytomolecules. Whereas, the standard drug donazepril has an ACE value of -365.13.

Inflammation Biomarkers

Neutrophils, the first defense molecules that come to the site of action, play an essential role in the pathogenesis of inflammation. These molecules release ROS, chemokines and protease enzymes by travelling to the extravascular space by binding to the vascular endothelial cells [64]. Stress leads to inflammation that causes damage to normal tissues and matrix proteins. In case of inflammation, the major targets that are involved include cyclooxygenase-2 (COX) and lipooxygenase (LOX). These phytomolecules act on these molecules to inhibit their action at the site of inflammation to resolve it [65]. Fig. (**4**) depicts the SAR studies of COX2 with lead phytobioactives and the results have been tabulated in Table **3**. Further, Fig. (**5**) depicts the SAR studies of LOX with lead phytobioactives and the results have been presented in Table **4**.

Table 3. Docking sites and there atomic contact energy values for inflammation disorder.

Name of the Biomarker	Name of the Compound	Details of H-bond Interaction	Atomic Contact Energy (ACE) Values	Amino Acid Residues on Docked Domains
		No. of Bond		
COX2 (Cyclooxygenase-2) (1CX2)	β-sitosterol	0	-348.50	Asn 34, Cys 36, Cys 37, Cys 41, Arg 44, Glu 46, Cys 47, Tyr 130 , Gly 135, Leu 152, Pro 153, Ala 156
	Catechin	17	-436.76	Glu 322, Trp 323, Glu 326, Gln 327, Ser 548, Thr 549, Asn 34, Pro 35, Cys 36, Asn 39, Glu 46, Cys 47, Met 48, Ser 49, His 133, Tyr 134, Gly 135, Tyr 136, Pro 153, Val 155, Ala 156, Asp 157
	Lupeol	1	-329.21	Cys 36, Asn 39, Cys 41, Arg 44, Gly 45, Cys 47, Gly 135, Pro 153, Ala 156, Gln 461, Glu 465
	Naringenin	2	-242.90	Leu 352, Ser 353, Tyr 355, Tyr 385, Trp 387, Ala 527, Leu 531
	Indomethacin	1	-280.13	Gln 192, Tyr 348, Val 349, Leu 352, Ser 353, Leu 359, Tyr 385, Val 523

The results exhibited catechin had the highest ACE value of -436.76 among the top 4 phytomolecules. Whereas, the standard drug indomethacin has an ACE value of -280.13.

Ulcer Biomarkers

Chronic inflammation in the stomach or intestine leads to the formation of ulcers that is the break in the mucosal lining caused by *Helicobacter pylori* infection [66]. This infection causes gastritis that predominantly leads to disease pattern cancer. While cancer is a disease that is life-threatening and cannot be cured except for some cancer types. Sodium potassium ATPase also known as the energy producer, is responsible for the pathogenesis of ulcers [67]. ATPase that synthesizes ATP is inhibited, these phytomolecules may have the ability to treat ulcer by targeting ATPase. Fig. (**6**) depicts the SAR studies of ATPase with lead phytobioactives and the results have been tabulated in Table **5**.

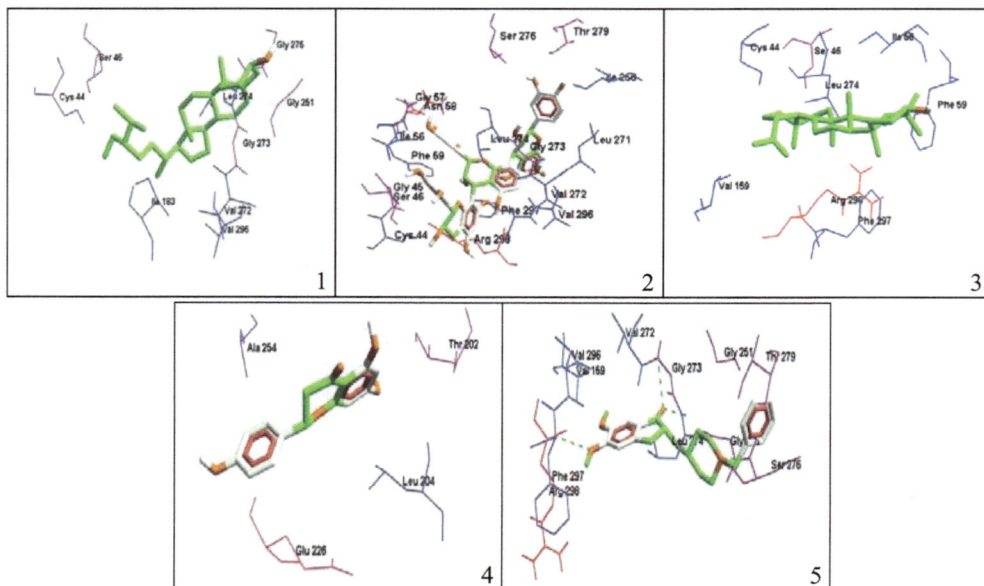

Fig. (3). (1) SOD and Catechin, **(2)** SOD and Naringenin, **((3)** SOD and Lupeol, **(4)** SOD and β-sitosterol **(5)** SOD and Donazepril.

Diabetic Biomarkers

Diabetes is a disorder where the body is unable to produce a sufficient amount of insulin for the metabolic processes. Type 2 diabetes is a major concern due to unhealthy lifestyle and stress [68]. Prolonged pathogenesis of diabetes leads to vascular complications including neuropathy, cardiovascular diseases, nephropathy and strokes. The pathways involved include the polyol pathway, hexosamine pathway, and mitogen-activated protein kinase pathway that lead to the over-expression of ROS causing pathogenesis of diabetic complications [69]. Targeting aldol reductase and acetyl CoA carboxylase-2 (ACC2) would ameliorate the disorder since these phytomolecules have potent medicinal value [70]. Fig. (**7**) depicts the SAR studies of Aldol reductase with lead phytobioactives and the results have been tabulated in Table **6**. Further, Fig. (**8**) depicts the SAR studies of Acetyl CoA carboxylase-2 with lead phytobioactives and the results have been tabulated in Table **7**.

Fig. (4). **(6)** COX2 and β-sitosterol, **(7)** COX2 and Catechin, **(8)** COX2 and Lupeol, **(9)** COX2 and Naringenin, **(10)** COX2 and Indomethacin.

Fig. (5). **(11)** LOX and β-sitosterol, **(12)** LOX and Catechin, **(13)** LOX and Lupeol, **(14)** LOX and Naringenin, **(15)** LOX and Indomethacin.

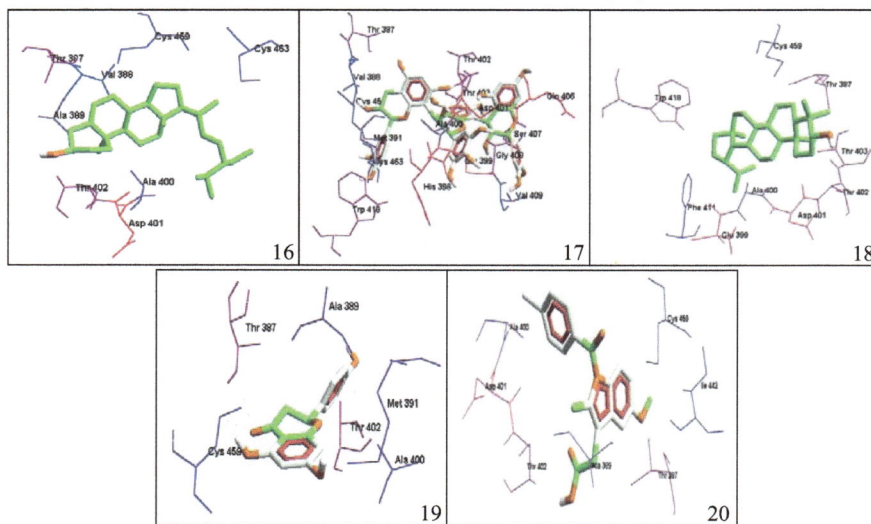

Fig. (6). (16) ATPase and β-sitosterol, **(17)**) ATPase and Catechin, **(18)** ATPase and Lupeol, **(19)** ATPase and Naringenin, **(20)** ATPase and Indomethacin.

Table 4. Docking sites and there atomic contact energy values for inflammation.

Name of the Biomarker	Name of the Compound	Details of H-bond Interaction	Atomic Contact Energy (ACE)	Amino Acid Residues on Docked Domains
		No. of Bond	Values	
LOX (Lipooxygenase) (1YGE)	β-sitosterol	1	-274.77	Val 126, Cys 127, Asn 128, Ser 129, Ile 142, Phe 143, Phe 144, Glu 165, Arg 182, Asp 243, Val 520, Tyr 525, Thr 529, Asp 768, Trp 772
	Catechin	1	-623.36	Val 126, Cys 127, Asn 128, Ser 129, Ile 142, Phe 143, Phe 144, Glu 165, Arg 182, Asp 243, Val 520, Tyr 525, Thr 529, Asp 768, Trp 772
	Lupeol	2	-205.86	Trp 772, Asp 243, Glu 244, Leu 246, Val 520, Thr 529, Pro 530, Arg 533, Asp 768
	Naringenin	3	-201.15	Val 126, Cys 127, Ser 129, Arg 141, Phe 143, Phe 144, Ala 145, Asn 146, Val 520, Lys 526, Trp 772
	Indomethacin	5	-143.98	Tyr 137, Lys 138, Ser 139, Val 140, Ser 168, Tyr 180, Asp 181, Ile 183

The results exhibited catechin had the highest ACE value of -623.36 among the top 4 phytomolecules. Whereas, the standard drug indomethacin has an ACE value of -280.13

Table 5. Docking sites and there atomic contact energy values for cancer.

Name of the Biomarker	Name of the Compound	Details of H-bond interaction	Atomic contact Energy (ACE)	Amino acid residues on docked domains
		No. of bond	Values	
Sodium potassium ATPase (1MO7)	β-sitosterol	0	-326.07	Thr 387, Val 388, Ala 389, Ala 400, Asp 401, Thr 402, Cys 459, Cys 463
	Catechin	23	-599.81	Thr 387, Val 388, Met 391, His 398, Glu 399, Ala 400, Asp 401, Thr 402, Thr 403, Gln 406, Ser 407, Gly 408, Val 409, Trp 418, Cys 459, Cys 463
	Lupeol	0	-295.47	Thr 387, Glu 399, Ala 400, Asp 401, Thr 402, Thr 403, Phe 411, Cys 459, Trp 418
	Naringenin	3	-199.40	Thr 387, Ala 389, Met 391, Ala 400, Thr 402, Cys 459
	Indomethacin	0	-224.25	Cys 459, Thr 387, Ala 389, Ala 400, Asp 401, Thr 402, Ile 442

The results exhibited catechin had the highest ACE value of -599.81 among the top 4 phytomolecules. Whereas, the standard drug indomethacin has an ACE value of -224.25

Fig. (7). (21) Aldol reductase and β-sitosterol, **(22)** Aldol reductase and Catechin, **(23)** Aldol reductase and Lupeol, **(24)** Aldol reductase and Naringenin, **(25)** Aldol reductase and Metformin.

Table 6. Docking sites and there atomic contact energy values for diabetes.

Name of the Biomarker	Name of the Compound	Details of H-bond Interaction	Atomic Contact Energy (ACE) Values	Amino Acid Residues on Docked Domains
		No. of Bond		
Aldol reductase (4JIR)	β-sitosterol	1	-349.72	Trp 20, His 110, Trp 111, Phe 122, Trp 219, Val 297, Cys 298, Ala 299, Leu 300, Leu 301
	Catechin	6	-482.42	Trp 20, Val 47, Tyr 48, His 110, Trp 111, Phe 122, Leu 124, Tyr 209, Ser 210, Arg 217, Pro 218, Trp 219, Cys 298, Leu 300, Leu 301, Ser 302
	Lupeol	0	-364.68	Trp 20, Tyr 48, Trp 79, His 110, Phe 122, Trp 219, Leu 300, Leu 301, Ser 302
	Naringenin	1	-213.95	Val 47, Trp 79, His 110, Phe 122, Trp 219, Cys 298, Leu 300
	Metformin	2	-114.19	Trp 20, Tyr 48, Ser 210, Ile 260, Lys 262

The results exhibited catechin had the highest ACE value of -482.42 among the top 4 phytomolecules. Whereas, the standard drug metformin has an ACE value of -114.19.

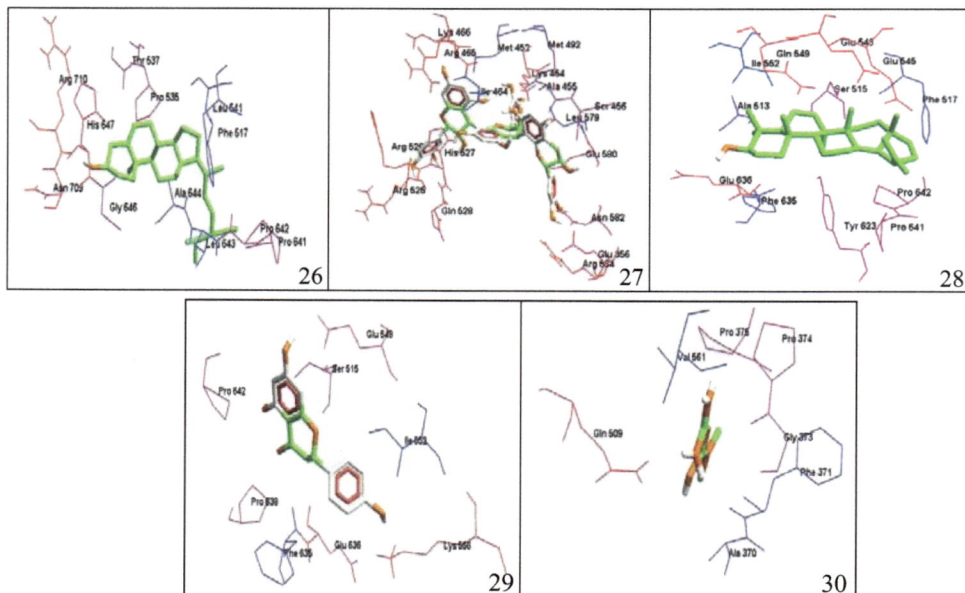

Fig. (8). (26) ACC2 and β-sitosterol, **(27)** ACC2 and Catechin, **(28)** ACC2 and Lupeol, **(29)** ACC2 and Naringenin, **(30)** ACC2 and Metformin.

Table 7. Docking sites and there atomic contact energy values for diabetes.

Name of the Biomarker	Name of the Compound	Details of H-bond Interaction	Atomic Contact Energy (ACE)	Amino Acid Residues on Docked Domains
		No. of Bond	Values	
ACC2 (Acetyl CoA carboxylase-2) (3JRW)	β-sitosterol	1	-298.14	Phe 517, Pro 535, Thr 537, Leu 541, Pro 641, Pro 642, Leu 643, Ala 644, Gly 646, His 647, Asn 709, Arg 710
	Catechin	13	-167.80	Glu 356, Met 452, Lys 454, Ala 455, Ser 456, Ile 464, Arg 465, Lys 466, Met 492, Arg 525, Arg 526, His 527, Leu 579, Glu 580, Gln 528, Arg 584, Asn 582
	Lupeol	0	-244.75	Pro 642, Ala 513, Ser 515, Phe 517, Glu 545, Glu 548, Gln 549, Ile 552, Tyr 623, Phe 635, Glu 636, Pro 641
	Naringenin	4	-167.50	Ser 515, Glu 548, Ile 552, Lys 556, Phe 635, Glu 636, Pro 638, Pro 642, Ser 515, Glu 548, Ile 552, Lys 556, Phe 635, Glu 636, Pro 638, Pro 642
	Metformin	2	-151.92	Ala 370, Phe 371, Gly 373, Pro 374, Pro 375, Gln 509, Val 561

The results exhibited β-sitosterol had the highest ACE value of -298.14 among the top 4 phytomolecules. Whereas, the standard drug metformin has an ACE value of -151.92.

Liver Biomarkers

Stress on an individual leads to depression, fatigue and many other complications where the individual takes up alcohol to relieve the stress accumulated. This leads to a major disorder of the liver called liver cirrhosis where 'cirrhosis' meaning the tan color of the liver. The condition may also occur in non-alcoholic individuals called the fatty liver disease. To determine how healthy the liver is, the liver enzymes are measured including alkaline phosphatase, aspartate amino transferase and alanine amino transferase. Therefore targeting these enzymes of the liver would ameliorate the disorder [71]. Fig. (**9**) depicts the SAR studies of Alkaline phosphatase with lead phytobioactives and the results have been tabulated in Table **8**. Further, Fig. (**10**) depicts the SAR studies of Aspartate amino transferase with lead phytobioactives and the results have been tabulated in Table **9**.

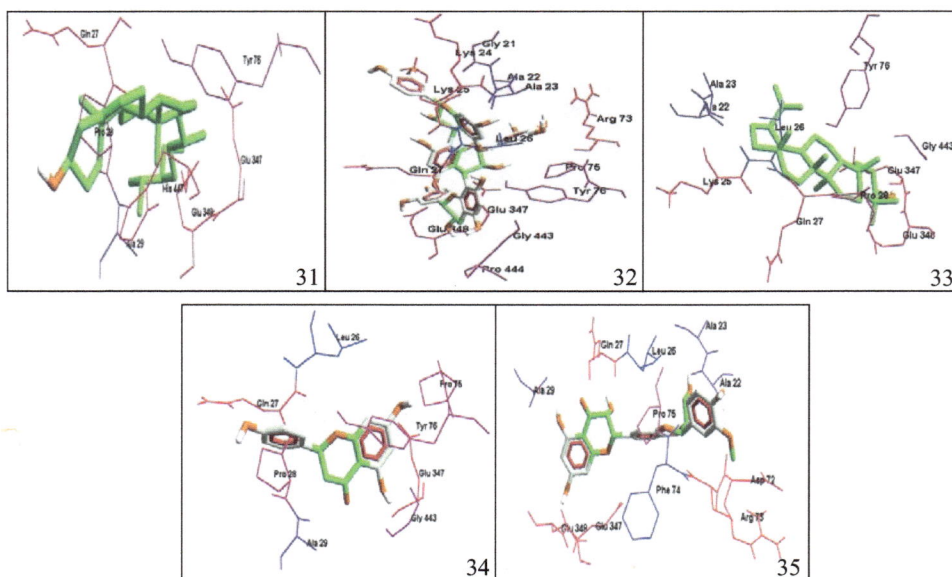

Fig. (9). **(31)** ALP and β-sitosterol, **(32)** ALP and Catechin, **(33)** ALP and Lupeol, **(34)** ALP and Naringenin, **(35)** ALP and Silymarin.

Table 8. Docking sites and there atomic contact energy values for liver disorders.

Name of the Biomarker	Name of the Compound	Details of H-bond Interaction	Atomic Contact Energy (ACE)	Amino Acid Residues on Docked Domains
		No. of Bond	Values	
Alkaline phosphatase (ALP) (1EW2)	**β-sitosterol**	0	-332.82	Gln 27, Pro 28, Ala 29, Tyr 76, Glu 347, Glu 348, His 447
	Catechin	16	-428.45	Gly 21, Ala 22, Ala 23, Lys 24, Lys 25, Leu 26, Gln 27, Arg 73, Pro 75, Tyr 76, Glu 347, Glu 348, Gly 443, Pro 444
	Lupeol	1	-426.72	Ala 22, Ala 23, Lys 25, Leu 26, Gln 27, Pro 28, Tyr 76, Glu 347, Glu 348, Gly 443
	Naringenin	5	-185.41	Leu 26, Gln 27, Pro 28, Ala 29, Pro 75, Tyr 76, Glu 347, Gly 443
	Silymarin	5	-273.61	Glu 348, Ala 22, Ala 23, Leu 26, Gln 27, Ala 29, Asp 72, Arg 73, Phe 74, Pro 75, Glu 347

The results exhibited β-sitosterol had the highest ACE value of -428.45 among the top 4 phytomolecules. Whereas, the standard drug silymarin has an ACE value of -273.61.

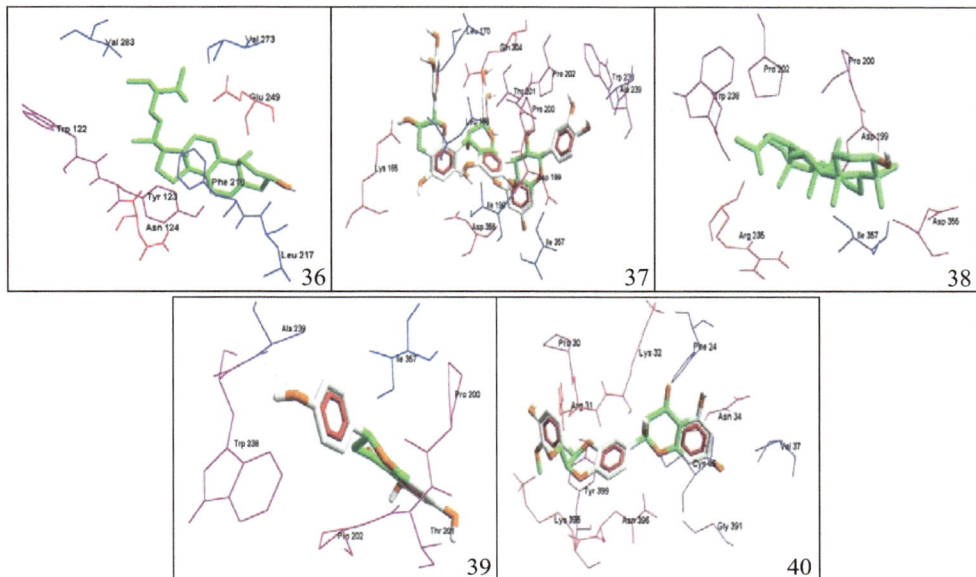

Fig. (10). **(36)** AST and β-sitosterol, **(37)** AST and Catechin, **(38)** AST and Lupeol, **(39)** AST and Naringenin, **(40)** AST and Silymarin.

Table 9. Docking sites and there atomic contact energy values for liver disorders.

Name of the Biomarker	Name of the Compound	Details of H-bond Interaction	Atomic Contact Energy (ACE) Values	Amino Acid Residues on Docked Domains
		No. of Bond		
Aspartate amino transferase (AST) (3WZF)	β-sitosterol	2	-257.42	Trp 122, Tyr 123, Asn 124, Leu 217, Phe 218, Glu 249, Val 273, Val 283
	Catechin	7	-302.16	Lys 165, Leu 168, Leu 170, Ile 198, Asp 199, Pro 200, Thr 201, Pro 202, Gln 204, Trp 238, Ala 239, Asp 355, Ile 357
	Lupeol	1	-275.45	Asp 199, Pro 200, Pro 202, Arg 235, Trp 238, Asp 355, Ile 357
	Naringenin	2	-172.90	Pro 200, Thr 201, Pro 202, Trp 238, Ala 239, Ile 357
	Silymarin	4	-281.44	Phe 24, Pro 30, Arg 31, Lys 32, Asn 34, Val 37, Cys 45, Gly 391, Lys 395, Asn 396, Tyr 399

The results exhibited β-sitosterol had the highest ACE value of -302.16 among the top 4 phytomolecules. Whereas, the standard drug Silymarin has an ACE value of -281.44.

Venom Biomarkers

Venoms produced by snakes are basically of three types, including myotoxic (that affects the cardiac muscles), hemotoxic (that affects the red blood cells) and neurotoxic (that affects the nervous system) [47]. This venom that is a cocktail of proteins and lipids interacts with the proteins and lipids present in the body and degrades them causing damage leading to death. The venomous proteins and lipids act on enzymes in the body majorly phophodiesterase, acetyl-choline esterase and phospholipase A_2 [44] therefore targeting these molecules and protecting them using these phytomolecules would be of therapeutic value. Fig. (**11**) depicts the SAR studies of Acetyl choline esterase and Phosphodiesterase with lead phytobioactives and the results have been tabulated in Table **10**.

Fig. (11). (**41**) AChE and β-sitosterol, (**42**) AChE and Catechin, (**43**) AChE and Lupeol, (**44**) AChE and Naringenin, (**45**) Phosphodiesterase and β-sitosterol, (**46**) Phosphodiesterase and Catechin, (**47**) Phosphodiesterase and Lupeol, (**48**) Phosphodiesterase and Naringenin.

Table 10. Docking sites and there atomic contact energy values for liver disorders.

Name of the Biomarker	Name of the Compound	Details of H-bond Interaction	Atomic Contact Energy (ACE) Values	Amino Acid Residues on Docked Domains
		No. of Bond		
Acetyl choline esterase (AChE) (3LII)	β-sitosterol	0	-341.43	Trp 86, Gly 121, Tyr 124, Ser 125, Ser 203, Trp 286, Phe 297, Phe 338, Tyr 341
	Catechin	10	-441.56	Tyr 341, Tyr 72, Thr 75, Leu 76, Tyr 124, Gln 279, Asn 283, Trp 286, His 287, Ser 293, Val 294, Phe 295, Arg 296, Phe 297, Tyr 337
	Lupeol	0	-315.70	Asp 74, Trp 86, Gly 121, Tyr 124, Ser 125, Glu 202, Trp 286, Phe 297, Tyr 337, Tyr 341
	Naringenin	1	-189.09	Tyr 341, Asp 74, Trp 86, Tyr 124, Val 294, Phe 297, Tyr 337
Phosphodiesterase (1WOJ)	β-sitosterol	0	-270.17	Val 322, Leu 168, Tyr 169, Thr 233, Lys 235, Phe 236, Val 294, Arg 308, His 310, Ala 321
	Catechin	8	-441.36	Gly 379, Leu 168, Phe 173, Arg 225, Pro 226, Pro 227, Val 229, His 231, His 310, Thr 312, Ala 321, Thr 375, Gly 376, Tyr 377
	Lupeol	0	-249.41	Val 322, His 231, Thr 233, Phe 236, Val 294, Ala 321
	Naringenin	2	-175.56	Ala 321, Tyr 169, Phe 173, Arg 225, Val 229, His 231, Thr 312, Cys 315

The results exhibited Catechin had the highest ACE value of -441.56 with the target AChE and -441.36 with phosphodiesterase among the top 4 phytomolecules, respectively. From all the above-obtained results, it is found that catechin is the top one potent phytomolecule that has the maximum activity in all the cases. Further experiments need to be carried out to authenticate its ability in treating the diseases.

TAMARIND PROCESSING AND PRODUCTS

Processing and Preservation

Once the tamarind tree is fully grown, it yields about 180–225 kg of fruits per season [72]. The total yield of tamarind pods per tree is estimated at approximately 175 kg and 70 kg pulp for processing from per tree in India. Residual seeds, fiber and other foreign matter, can be separated by pulping it with shelled tamarind fruits with a small amount of water and passing them through a pulper [73]. University of Agricultural Sciences (UAS) Bangalore, India has designed a tamarind dehuller machine. This machine capacity for hulling is 500 kg per hour, with 80 per-cent efficiency for large fruits and small fruits of 58 per-cent. On the basis of the report, it was observed that tamarind fruit undergoes post-harvest physiological and chemical changes. Processing within one week of harvest maximal amount of yield can be obtained from tamarind [74]. The pulp is preserved by pressing in large quantities and sold in markets and retail shops for required quantities in several tamarind-growing countries. For packing and transportation purposes the pulp is made free from fiber and seeds then usually mixed with 10% salt beaten down with mallets to exclude air and packed in gunny bags, lined with palm-leaf matting [75]. In India, the pulp is stored in earthenware jars and preserved by rolling it in salt as a preservative and exposed to moisture [76]. Whereas Java is an island of Indonesia like java, the pulp is stored in stone jars and preserved by salting and rolled into balls, steamed and sun-dried, then exposed to moisture for a week before packing. In Thailand, the pulp is stored in plastic bags to exclude air preserved by adding salt and compressing. In Sri Lanka, the harvested pods are sun-dried for 5-7 days in order to bring all the immature fruits to matured, fully ripen stage. Later, the pulp is separated along with seeds is then dried for the next 3-4 days to eliminate excess moisture and avoid mold growth by adding salt and preserved in clay pots [77]. The freshly extracted pulp is light brown in color. The research conducted at CFTRI (Central Food Technological Research Institute) Mysore, India found that without treatment, the pulp can be preserved for 6-8months, if stored in air-tight containers at cool and dry place [76]. According to Food and Agricultural Organization (FAO) (1989) [72], as per reports of FAO (1989), spoilage starts when the tamarind is continuous storage for long periods under extremes of temperature and humidity, which leads to color change from brown or yellowish-brown to black. Good quality tamarind is prepared by CFTRI by improving the process of paste preparation which is free from seeds, fibrous and foreign matters. The cleaned pulp is processed using heat, then it is coarsely grinded, later reprocessed to minimize the moisture content to obtain a good quality of tamarind paste [78]. In Thailand, a method of sweet tamarind processing is documented, where fruits are steamed for 5 minutes, then dried in a hot air oven at 80°C for 2 hours and stored in a plastic bag at room temperature. Thus, by this method, the fruits can be preserved for four months without any deterioration in quality [79]. In various experiments, it is found that cold storage of tamarind pulp at different temperatures increases shelf-life of the product and freshly harvested, deseeded tamarind pulp can be stored for up to 330 days under refrigeration at 4±2°C with vacuum packed in 800-gauge poly bags without any color deterioration in the pulp right from the initial stage of storage [80].

Tamarind Products

Pulp

In India, tamarind is used in many different dishes, whereas tamarind pulp is the main source for tamarind. It plays an important role in souring curries, sauces, chutneys and certain beverages. Immature green pods are commonly eaten by children and adults by dipped in salt as a snack and also used as food seasoning for cooked rice, meat products, fish, delicious sauces of duck, waterfowl and geese. It is also used as seafood in making pickles out of fish which is considered a great delicacy in coastal areas and throughout the greater part of India [77]. Wine like beverages can also be prepared from tamarind fruit as raw material [81]. In Sri Lanka (Country neighboring India in the Indian Ocean), tamarind is widely used in different dishes like pickles, chutneys and an alternate to lime [82]. In Egypt during summer, sour drinks and similar lemon-flavored drinks are made using tamarind which has great demand in the Middle East. Likewise, in Mexico, different drinks are made which are popularly called agua fresca (refreshing water) or 'aguadetamrindo' which is sometimes turned into frozen fruit ices. Here, tamarind is also used as a snack, dried, salted or candied (*e.g.*, Pulparindo). The Philippines also use tamarind in making sweets and its leaves are used in the famous recipes of sinigang soup. In Guadeloupe, tamarind fruits which are fully ripped are used in the preparation of jam and syrup, whereas Nigeria tamarind is used in preparing their breakfast, as it is added to the traditional porridge known as pap or kununtsamiya. It is mainly used in the preparation of sauces to give a sour flavor, for popular pad Thai from Thailand, or in gravy for Assam fish in Singapore and Malaya [83].

Juice Concentrate

There is a great market for tamarind juice in India and aboard [74]. By boiling it with water, all the water-soluble compounds are extracted from fruit pulp, then concentrated to about 65–70% solids and packed in suitable containers. The product obtained is viscous and sets to the consistency of jam on cooling. When compared to sucrose solutions, tamarind juice concentrate is more viscous [84]. Thus, it has been reported that spiced sauces and beverages can also be prepared using pulp [75]. CFTRI formulated the approximate composition of concentrate as, total tartaric acid 13%; invert sugars 50%; pectin 2%; protein 3%; cellulosic material 2%; and moisture 30%, respectively.

Tamarind-Mango Squash

Once tamarind is procured, cleaned and deseeded, it is pretreated before use. It is soaked in water at 1:1:5 ratios, boiled to 100°C, then cooled to crush, later it is sieved to obtain the pulp. This pulp serves in the preparation of mango squash called tamarind mango squash, which is prepared out of 30% pulp, sugar concentration of 46°Brix and Potassium Metabi-sulphate as a preservative. It is stored in sterilized bottles and capped airtightly. For reconstitution, it is diluted in the ratio of 1:4 juice and water before serving [85].

Tamarind Jam

Tamarind pulp is used for the preparation of jam by blending with different levels of 50 percent mango pulp. Extracted tamarind pulp is mixed with sugar (175 percent) and heated to 100°C. The pectin is used as a gelling agent and added in a concentration of 1 per-cent. The mixture is boiled till the end-point is achieved. The hot mixture is filled in sterile bottles and allowed to cool. Post cooling the bottles are sealed stored and transported [86].

Spiced Tamarind Beverage

Adeola and Aworh reformed the method of tamarind beverage preparation; here, the pulp was separated manually from shells, seeds and other foreign matters. Tamarind pulp is mixed with water in the ratio of 1:175; spices like, ginger 0.6%; clove 0.4%; and sugar of 27.5% are added and the obtained juice is filtered using muslin cloth which is folded to form four layers. This clarified beverage is mixed with 100 mg sodium benzoate per 100 mL concentration. Then, this beverage is stored in glass bottles which are sterilized, corked and pasteurized at 95°C for 8 min. This tamarind beverage is refrigerated (4–10°C) and it has a shelf life of 4 months [88].

Food Colorant

In Japan tamarind brown color is extracted naturally from tamarind as a food colorant [78]. The main pigments present are leucoanthocyanidin and anthocyanin [76, 89]. Natural and attractive red color of tamarind is imparted to variety of foods like; curries, jam, jelly and many others in traditional foods. Natural red colorant which is extracted from red tamarind is very widely used in the food industry. It has many health benefits and reduces environmental burden [89].

Quality Aspects of Tamarind

Maintaining the quality of the tamarind products is real challenge due to various aspects like seed, fiber, moisture content and rind contents. It is very frequent to be adulterated with foreign matter which could be organic or inorganic source. Due to lack of post harvest practices adulteration is the main reason, it could be accidental or purposefully [90]. There are some important quality standards specified by Directorate of Marketing and Inspection, Institute Governing Standards, Bureau of Indian Standards (BIS) for variety of tamarind derivatives like seedless tamarind, dry tamarind and tamarind seed [91]. The Indian standards specified concentrates of tamarind juice (IS 5955), pulp (IS 6364), kernel oil (IS 9587: 1980) and kernel powder (IS 189: 1977), IS 511: 1962.

CONCLUSION

It can be concluded saying that the most valuable and commonly used part of tamarind tree is the fruit having a great economic value. The pulp constitutes 30 to 50 percent of the ripe fruit, the shell and fiber account for 11 to 30 percent and the seed about 25-40 per cent. Tamarind is commonly used as a health remedy throughout Asia, Africa and the Americas for various disorders and ailments. Tamarind products, leaves, fruits and seeds have been extensively used in Indian Ayurvedic medicine and traditional African medicine. In these systems of medicine the molecular mechanism of action of the plant cannot be determined therefore studying the mechanism of action of the phytomolecules would advance the therapeutic value. But due to its economic value one of major concern is tamarind is reported to have been adulterated with foreign matter which is both organic and inorganic in nature, due to poor post-harvest management practices including processing. With better post harvesting procedures, techniques and tools the number of adulterants could be reduced them by enhancing the pure availability of tamarind products. The storage conditions, hygiene and proper process guidelines by AGMARK and other Agri-produce agencies will help establishing quality norms of tamarind and its products. Tamarind food products apart from just as an ingredient in cooking there are many beverages, snacks been prepared and will be available in market in near future. Proper manufacturing conditions and transportation facilities like cold chain logistics will propel this sector to a great extent. The ultimate intent is to have a holistic approach to popularize the concept of making food as medicine to address various clinical complications with the power of spices and herbs for transforming Devil's tree with sour date to God's medicine with sweet cure.

ABBREVIATIONS

ACC2 Acetyl CoA Carboxylase-2

ACE Atomic Contact Energy

AChE Acetyl choline esterase

ALP Alkaline phosphatase

AST Aspartate amino transferase

BIS Bureau of Indian Standards

CFTRI Central Food Technological Research Institute

COX Cyclooxygenase-2

FAO Food and Agricultural Organization

INH Isoniazid

LOX Lipooxygenase

PDB Protein Data Bank

PZA Pyraziamide

RIF Rifampicin

RNS Reactive nitrogen species

ROS Reactive oxygen species

SAR Structure-activity relationship

SGOT Serum glutamate oxaloacetate transaminase

SGPT Serum glutamate pyruvate transaminase

SOD Superoxide Dismutase

TB Tuberculosis

TGF-β Tumor Growth Factor- β

UAS University of Agricultural Sciences

VEGF Vascular Endothelial Growth Factor

CONSENT FOR PUBLICATION

Not applicable.

CONFLICT OF INTEREST

The authors confirm that the contents of this chapter have no conflict of interest.

ACKNOWLEDGEMENTS

Pankaj Satapathy would like to thank DST-KSTePS, GoK, for providing DST Ph.D. fellowship (LIF-09-2018-19). Ms. Aishwarya. T. Devi would like to thank the Indian Council of Medical Research (ICMR) for the award of Senior Research Fellow (SRF) Award Letter Number - File no.5/3/8/55/ITR-F/2018-ITR dated 11.6.2018. All authors thank the Hon'ble Vice-Chancellor, JSS Science and Technology University, Principal, SJCE, Mysore for his encouragement and JSS research foundation for their constant inspiration. Mr. Avinash MG would like to thank the Indian Council of Medical Research (ICMR) for the award of Senior Research Fellow (SRF) Award Letter Number - File no. AMR/Fellowship/ 17/2019 ECD-II dated 28.6.2019. FZ sincerely acknowledges the University Grants Commission (UGC), Govt. of India, New Delhi, for awarding Raman Post-Doctoral Fellowship to USA (Ref No. F.5-97/2014 (IC) FD dairy no: 6725). Further, we extend our gratitude towards the management and office bearers of Dayananda Sagar University, Bengaluru, Karnataka, India, for constant inspiration, motivation, and encouragement to pursue scientific research.

REFERENCES

[1] Havinga RM, Hartl A, Putscher J, Prehsler S, Buchmann C, Vogl CR. *Tamarindus indica* L. (Fabaceae): patterns of use in traditional African medicine. J Ethnopharmacol 2010; 127(3): 573-88. [http://dx.doi.org/10.1016/j.jep.2009.11.028] [PMID: 19963055]

[2] El-Siddig K. Tamarind: Tamarindus indica. L. Crops for the Future 2006.

[3] National Research Council. Toward sustainable agricultural systems in the 21st century. National Academies Press. 2010.

[4] Morton JF, Dowling CF. Fruits of warm climates. Miami, FL: JF Morton 1987.

[5] Martinello F, Soares SM, Franco JJ, *et al.* Hypolipemic and antioxidant activities from *Tamarindus indica* L. pulp fruit extract in hypercholesterolemic hamsters. Food Chem Toxicol 2006; 44(6): 810-8. [http://dx.doi.org/10.1016/j.fct.2005.10.011] [PMID: 16330140]

[6] Thakur M, Bhargava S, Praznik W, Loeppert R, Dixit VK. Effect of *Chlorophytum Borivilianum* Santapau and Fernandes on sexual dysfunction in hyperglycemic male rats. Chin J Integr Med 2009; 15(6): 448-53. [http://dx.doi.org/10.1007/s11655-009-0448-6] [PMID: 20082251]

[7] Rasul N, Saleem B, Nawaz R. Preliminary phytochemical screening of four common plants of family *caesalpiniaceae*. Pak J Pharm Sci 1989; 2(1): 55-7. [PMID: 16414637]

[8] Coutiño-Rodríguez R, Hernández-Cruz P, Giles-Ríos H. Lectins in fruits having gastrointestinal activity: their participation in the hemagglutinating property of Escherichia coli O157:H7. Arch Med Res 2001; 32(4): 251-7. [http://dx.doi.org/10.1016/S0188-4409(01)00287-9] [PMID: 11440778]

[9] Kobayashi A, Adenan MI, Kajiyama S, Kanzaki H, Kawazu K. A cytotoxic principle of *Tamarindus indica*, di-n-butyl malate and the structure-activity relationship of its analogues. Z Natforsch C J Biosci 1996; 51(3-4): 233-42. [http://dx.doi.org/10.1515/znc-1996-3-415] [PMID: 8639230]

[10] Khanzada SK, Shaikh W, Sofia S, *et al.* Chemical constituents of *Tamarindus indica* L. medicinal plant in Sindh. Pak J Bot 2008; 40(6): 2553-9.

[11] Mishra RN. *Tamarindus indica* L: An Overview of Tree Improvement. InProc. 1997; 294.

[12] Ebifa-Othieno E, Mugisha A, Nyeko P, Kabasa JD. Knowledge, attitudes and practices in tamarind (*Tamarindus indica* L) use and conservation in Eastern Uganda. J Ethnobiol Ethnomed 2017; 13(1): 5.

[http://dx.doi.org/10.1186/s13002-016-0133-8] [PMID: 28109300]

[13]   Yalcin MM, Altinova AE, Ozkan C, *et al.* Thyroid malignancy risk of incidental thyroid nodules in patients with non-thyroid cancer. Acta Endocrinol (Bucur) 2016; 12(2): 185-90.
[http://dx.doi.org/10.4183/aeb.2016.185] [PMID: 31149085]

[14]   Alberti KG, Zimmet PZ. Definition, diagnosis and classification of diabetes mellitus and its complications. Part 1: diagnosis and classification of diabetes mellitus provisional report of a WHO consultation. Diabet Med 1998; 15(7): 539-53.
[http://dx.doi.org/10.1002/(SICI)1096-9136(199807)15:7<539::AID-DIA668>3.0.CO;2-S]   [PMID: 9686693]

[15]   Gokcel A, Karakose H, Ertorer EM, Tanaci N, Tutuncu NB, Guvener N. Effects of sibutramine in obese female subjects with type 2 diabetes and poor blood glucose control. Diabetes Care 2001; 24(11): 1957-60.
[http://dx.doi.org/10.2337/diacare.24.11.1957] [PMID: 11679464]

[16]   Bhadoriya SS, Ganeshpurkar A, Bhadoriya RPS, Sahu SK, Patel JR. Antidiabetic potential of polyphenolic-rich fraction of *Tamarindus indica* seed coat in alloxan-induced diabetic rats. J Basic Clin Physiol Pharmacol 2018; 29(1): 37-45.
[http://dx.doi.org/10.1515/jbcpp-2016-0193] [PMID: 28888089]

[17]   Ong KW, Hsu A, Song L, Huang D, Tan BK. Polyphenols-rich *Vernonia amygdalina* shows anti-diabetic effects in streptozotocin-induced diabetic rats. J Ethnopharmacol 2011; 133(2): 598-607.
[http://dx.doi.org/10.1016/j.jep.2010.10.046] [PMID: 21035531]

[18]   Ahmad N, Mukhtar H. Green tea polyphenols and cancer: biologic mechanisms and practical implications. Nutr Rev 1999; 57(3): 78-83.
[http://dx.doi.org/10.1111/j.1753-4887.1999.tb06927.x] [PMID: 10101921]

[19]   Noor R, Akhter S, Rahman F, Munshi SK, Kamal SM, Feroz F. Frequency of extensively drug-resistant tuberculosis (XDR-TB) among re-treatment cases in NIDCH, Dhaka, Bangladesh. J Infect Chemother 2013; 19(2): 243-8.
[http://dx.doi.org/10.1007/s10156-012-0490-8] [PMID: 23053506]

[20]   Ernst JD, Trevejo-Nuñez G, Banaiee N. Genomics and the evolution, pathogenesis, and diagnosis of tuberculosis. J Clin Invest 2007; 117(7): 1738-45.
[http://dx.doi.org/10.1172/JCI31810] [PMID: 17607348]

[21]   Awodele O, Akintonwa A, Osunkalu VO, Coker HA. Modulatory activity of antioxidants against the toxicity of Rifampicin *in vivo*. Rev Inst Med Trop São Paulo 2010; 52(1): 43-6.
[http://dx.doi.org/10.1590/S0036-46652010000100007] [PMID: 20305954]

[22]   Tasduq SA, Peerzada K, Koul S, Bhat R, Johri RK. Biochemical manifestations of anti-tuberculosis drugs induced hepatotoxicity and the effect of silymarin. Hepatol Res 2005; 31(3): 132-5.
[http://dx.doi.org/10.1016/j.hepres.2005.01.005] [PMID: 15777701]

[23]   Gautam R, Saklani A, Jachak SM. Indian medicinal plants as a source of antimycobacterial agents. J Ethnopharmacol 2007; 110(2): 200-34.
[http://dx.doi.org/10.1016/j.jep.2006.12.031] [PMID: 17276637]

[24]   Abbasi AM, Khan MA, Ahmad M, *et al.* Medicinal plants used for the treatment of jaundice and hepatitis based on socio-economic documentation. Afr J Biotechnol 2009; 8(8): 1643-50.

[25]   Amir M, Khan MA, Ahmad S, *et al.* Ameliorating effects of *Tamarindus indica* fruit extract on anti-tubercular drugs induced liver toxicity in rats. Nat Prod Res 2016; 30(6): 715-9.
[http://dx.doi.org/10.1080/14786419.2015.1039001] [PMID: 25978515]

[26]   Gonzalez LS III, Spencer JP. Aminoglycosides: a practical review. Am Fam Physician 1998; 58(8): 1811-20.
[PMID: 9835856]

[27]   Ullah N, Azam Khan M, Khan T, Ahmad W. Protective potential of *Tamarindus indica* against

gentamicin-induced nephrotoxicity. Pharm Biol 2014; 52(4): 428-34.
[http://dx.doi.org/10.3109/13880209.2013.840318] [PMID: 24417619]

[28]   Kotta S, Ansari SH, Ali J. Exploring scientifically proven herbal aphrodisiacs. Pharmacogn Rev 2013;
       7(13): 1-10.
       [PMID: 23922450]

[29]   Carlsen E, Giwercman A, Keiding N, Skakkebaek NE. Evidence for decreasing quality of semen
       during past 50 years. BMJ 1992; 305(6854): 609-13.
       [http://dx.doi.org/10.1136/bmj.305.6854.609] [PMID: 1393072]

[30]   Sk A, v J, G K, D U, P K. Declining semen quality among south Indian infertile men: A retrospective
       study. J Hum Reprod Sci 2008; 1(1): 15-8.
       [http://dx.doi.org/10.4103/0974-1208.38972] [PMID: 19562058]

[31]   Sharma R, Biedenharn KR, Fedor JM, Agarwal A. Lifestyle factors and reproductive health: taking
       control of your fertility. Reprod Biol Endocrinol 2013; 11(1): 66.
       [http://dx.doi.org/10.1186/1477-7827-11-66] [PMID: 23870423]

[32]   Bhadoriya SS, Ganeshpurkar A, Narwaria J, Rai G, Jain AP. *Tamarindus indica*: Extent of explored
       potential. Pharmacogn Rev 2011; 5(9): 73-81.
       [http://dx.doi.org/10.4103/0973-7847.79102] [PMID: 22096321]

[33]   De Caluwé E, Halamová K, Van Damme P. *Tamarindus indica* L. A review of traditional uses,
       phytochemistry and pharmacology. Afrika focus. 2010; 23: p. (1)53-83.

[34]   Dhiman P, Soni K, Singh S. Medicinal value of carom seeds–An overview. PharmaTutor 2014; 2(3):
       119-23.

[35]   Rai A, Das S, Chamallamudi MR, *et al.* Evaluation of the aphrodisiac potential of a chemically
       characterized aqueous extract of *Tamarindus indica* pulp. J Ethnopharmacol 2018; 210: 118-24.
       [http://dx.doi.org/10.1016/j.jep.2017.08.016] [PMID: 28830817]

[36]   Battin EE, Brumaghim JL. Antioxidant activity of sulfur and selenium: a review of reactive oxygen
       species scavenging, glutathione peroxidase, and metal-binding antioxidant mechanisms. Cell Biochem
       Biophys 2009; 55(1): 1-23.
       [http://dx.doi.org/10.1007/s12013-009-9054-7] [PMID: 19548119]

[37]   Bedi O, Bijjem KRV, Kumar P, Gauttam V. Herbal induced hepatoprotection and hepatotoxicity: A
       critical review. Indian J Physiol Pharmacol 2016; 60(1): 6-21.
       [PMID: 29953177]

[38]   Rodriguez Amado JR, Lafourcade Prada A, Escalona Arranz JC, *et al.* Antioxidant and
       Hepatoprotective Activity of a New Tablets Formulation from *Tamarindus indica* L Evidence-Based
       Complementary and Alternative Medicine 2016; 2016

[39]   Rodriguez-Amado JR, Lafourcade-Prada A, Arranz JC, Quevedo HM, Colarte AI, Carvalho JC.
       Optimization of a novel tablets formulation using D-optimal mixture design. Afr J Pharm Pharmacol
       2015; 9(14): 474-83.
       [http://dx.doi.org/10.5897/AJPP2014.4296]

[40]   Ismail M, Mariod A, Bagalkotkar G, Ling HS. Fatty acid composition and antioxidant activity of oils
       from two cultivars of Cantaloupe extracted by supercritical fluid extraction. Grasas Aceites 2010;
       61(1): 37-44.
       [http://dx.doi.org/10.3989/gya.053909]

[41]   Liolios CC, Sotiroudis GT, Chinou I. Fatty acids, sterols, phenols and antioxidant activity of *Phoenix
       theophrasti* fruits growing in Crete, Greece. Plant Foods Hum Nutr 2009; 64(1): 52-61.
       [http://dx.doi.org/10.1007/s11130-008-0100-1] [PMID: 19030994]

[42]   Sharma SK, Chappuis F, Jha N, Bovier PA, Loutan L, Koirala S. Impact of snake bites and
       determinants of fatal outcomes in southeastern Nepal. Am J Trop Med Hyg 2004; 71(2): 234-8.
       [http://dx.doi.org/10.4269/ajtmh.2004.71.234] [PMID: 15306717]

[43]   Bawaskar HS. Snake venoms and antivenoms: critical supply issues. J Assoc Physicians India 2004; 52: 11-3.
       [PMID: 15633710]

[44]   Brunda G, Sashidhar RB. Epidemiological profile of snake-bite cases from Andhra Pradesh using immunoanalytical approach. Indian J Med Res 2007; 125(5): 661-8.
       [PMID: 17642502]

[45]   Mors WB, Nascimento MC, Pereira BM, Pereira NA. Plant natural products active against snake bite--the molecular approach. Phytochemistry 2000; 55(6): 627-42.
       [http://dx.doi.org/10.1016/S0031-9422(00)00229-6] [PMID: 11130675]

[46]   Dey A, De JN. Traditional use of plants against snakebite in Indian subcontinent: a review of the recent literature. Afr J Tradit Complement Altern Med 2011; 9(1): 153-74.
       [http://dx.doi.org/10.4314/ajtcam.v9i1.20] [PMID: 23983332]

[47]   Pawar S, Patil DA. Ethnomedicinal uses of barks in Jalgaon district. Natural Product Radiance 2007; 6(4): 341-6.

[48]   Aird SD. Ophidian envenomation strategies and the role of purines. Toxicon 2002; 40(4): 335-93.
       [http://dx.doi.org/10.1016/S0041-0101(01)00232-X] [PMID: 11738231]

[49]   Shirwaikar A, Rajendran K, Bodla R, Kumar CD. Neutralization potential of *Viper russelli russelli* (Russell's viper) venom by ethanol leaf extract of Acalypha indica. J Ethnopharmacol 2004; 94(2-3): 267-73.
       [http://dx.doi.org/10.1016/j.jep.2004.05.010] [PMID: 15325729]

[50]   Ushanandini S, Nagaraju S, Harish Kumar K, *et al.* The anti-snake venom properties of *Tamarindus indica* (leguminosae) seed extract. Phytother Res 2006; 20(10): 851-8.
       [http://dx.doi.org/10.1002/ptr.1951] [PMID: 16847999]

[51]   Ramu R, S Shirahatti P, S NS, Zameer F, Bl D, M N NP. Correction: Assessment of *In Vivo* Antidiabetic Properties of Umbelliferone and Lupeol Constituents of Banana (Musa sp. var. Nanjangud Rasa Bale) Flower in Hyperglycaemic Rodent Model. PLoS One 2016; 11(7): e0160048.
       [http://dx.doi.org/10.1371/journal.pone.0160048] [PMID: 27438346]

[52]   Ramu R, Shirahatti PS, Anilakumar KR, *et al.* Assessment of nutritional quality and global antioxidant response of banana (Musa sp. CV. Nanjangud Rasa Bale) pseudostem and flower. Pharmacognosy Res 2017; 9 (Suppl. 1): S74-83.
       [http://dx.doi.org/10.4103/pr.pr_67_17] [PMID: 29333047]

[53]   Ramu R, Shirahatti PS, Zameer F, Prasad MN. Investigation of antihyperglycaemic activity of banana (Musa sp. var. Nanjangud rasa bale) pseudostem in normal and diabetic rats. J Sci Food Agric 2015; 95(1): 165-73.
       [http://dx.doi.org/10.1002/jsfa.6698] [PMID: 24752944]

[54]   Higdon JV, Frei B. Tea catechins and polyphenols: health effects, metabolism, and antioxidant functions. Crit Rev Food Sci Nutr 2003; 43(1): 89-143.
       [http://dx.doi.org/10.1080/10408690390826464]

[55]   Takanashi K, Suda M, Matsumoto K, *et al.* Epicatechin oligomers longer than trimers have anti-cancer activities, but not the catechin counterparts. Sci Rep 2017; 7(1): 7791.
       [http://dx.doi.org/10.1038/s41598-017-08059-x] [PMID: 28798415]

[56]   Hernández-Aquino E, Muriel P. Beneficial effects of naringenin in liver diseases: Molecular mechanisms. World J Gastroenterol 2018; 24(16): 1679-707.
       [http://dx.doi.org/10.3748/wjg.v24.i16.1679] [PMID: 29713125]

[57]   Den Hartogh DJ, Tsiani E. Antidiabetic properties of naringenin: a citrus fruit polyphenol. Biomolecules 2019; 9(3): 99.
       [http://dx.doi.org/10.3390/biom9030099] [PMID: 30871083]

[58] Zhang F, Dong W, Zeng W, *et al.* Naringenin prevents TGF-β1 secretion from breast cancer and suppresses pulmonary metastasis by inhibiting PKC activation. Breast Cancer Res 2016; 18(1): 38.
[http://dx.doi.org/10.1186/s13058-016-0698-0] [PMID: 27036297]

[59] Frabasile S, Koishi AC, Kuczera D, *et al.* The citrus flavanone naringenin impairs dengue virus replication in human cells. Sci Rep 2017; 7: 41864.
[http://dx.doi.org/10.1038/srep41864] [PMID: 28157234]

[60] Ke JY, Cole RM, Hamad EM, *et al.* Citrus flavonoid, naringenin, increases locomotor activity and reduces diacylglycerol accumulation in skeletal muscle of obese ovariectomized mice. Mol Nutr Food Res 2016; 60(2): 313-24.
[http://dx.doi.org/10.1002/mnfr.201500379] [PMID: 26573879]

[61] Thomsen R, Christensen MH. MolDock: a new technique for high-accuracy molecular docking. J Med Chem 2006; 49(11): 3315-21.
[http://dx.doi.org/10.1021/jm051197e] [PMID: 16722650]

[62] Schüttelkopf AW, van Aalten DM. PRODRG: a tool for high-throughput crystallography of protein-ligand complexes. Acta Crystallogr D Biol Crystallogr 2004; 60(Pt 8): 1355-63.
[http://dx.doi.org/10.1107/S0907444904011679] [PMID: 15272157]

[63] Landis GN, Tower J. Superoxide dismutase evolution and life span regulation. Mech Ageing Dev 2005; 126(3): 365-79.
[http://dx.doi.org/10.1016/j.mad.2004.08.012] [PMID: 15664623]

[64] Yasui K, Baba A. Therapeutic potential of superoxide dismutase (SOD) for resolution of inflammation. Inflamm Res 2006; 55(9): 359-63.
[http://dx.doi.org/10.1007/s00011-006-5195-y] [PMID: 17122956]

[65] Seibert K, Masferrer JL. Role of inducible cyclooxygenase (COX-2) in inflammation. Receptor 1994; 4(1): 17-23.
[PMID: 8038702]

[66] Shiotani A, Graham DY. Pathogenesis and therapy of gastric and duodenal ulcer disease. Med Clin North Am 2002; 86(6): 1447-1466, viii.
[http://dx.doi.org/10.1016/S0025-7125(02)00083-4] [PMID: 12510460]

[67] Graham DY. History of Helicobacter pylori, duodenal ulcer, gastric ulcer and gastric cancer. World J Gastroenterol 2014; 20(18): 5191-204.
[http://dx.doi.org/10.3748/wjg.v20.i18.5191] [PMID: 24833849]

[68] DeFronzo RA. Pathogenesis of type 2 diabetes mellitus. Med Clin North Am 2004; 88(4): 787-835, ix.
[http://dx.doi.org/10.1016/j.mcna.2004.04.013] [PMID: 15308380]

[69] Adeshara KA, Diwan AG, Tupe RS. G Diwan A, S Tupe R. Diabetes and complications: cellular signaling pathways, current understanding and targeted therapies. Curr Drug Targets 2016; 17(11): 1309-28.
[http://dx.doi.org/10.2174/1389450117666151209124007] [PMID: 26648059]

[70] Tang WH, Martin KA, Hwa J. Aldose reductase, oxidative stress, and diabetic mellitus. Front Pharmacol 2012; 3: 87.
[http://dx.doi.org/10.3389/fphar.2012.00087] [PMID: 22582044]

[71] Bendtsen F, Larsen FS, Ott P, Vilstrup H. [Cirrhosis of the liver]. Ugeskr Laeger 2014; 176(4): V02130126.
[PMID: 25095867]

[72] Prevention of Post-harvest Losses: Fruits, Vegetables and Root Crops, FAO Training Series No 17/2. Rome: FAO 1989.

[73] Benero JR, Rodríguez AJ, de Rivera AC. A Mechanical Method Fob Extracting Tamarind Pulp. J Agric Univ P R 1972; 56(2): 185-6.

[74]   Rao YS, Mathew KM. Tamarind In Handbook of Herbs and Spices. Woodhead Publishing 2012; p. 512-533.

[75]   Patil SJ, Nadagouder BS. Industrial products from *Tamarindus indica*. Proc Nat Sym on Tamarindus indica L 1997; 151-5..

[76]   Shankaracharya NB. Tamarind-chemistry, technology and uses-a critical appraisal. J Food Sci Technol 1998; 35(3): 193-208.

[77]   El-Siddig K, Gunasena HP, Prasad BA, *et al.* Tamarind (*Tamaridus Indica* L.). Southampton, UK: International Centre for Underutilized Crops. 2006.

[78]   Anon. . CSIR News 2003; 53(16): 30. a [August.].

[79]   Sambaiah K, Srinivasan K. Effect of cumin, cinnamon, ginger, mustard and tamarind in induced hypercholesterolemic rats. Nahrung 1991; 35(1): 47-51.
[http://dx.doi.org/10.1002/food.19910350112] [PMID: 1865890]

[80]   Nagalakshmi S, Chezhiyan N. Influence of type of packaging and storage conditions on Tamarind (*Tamarindus indica*) pulp quality. Journal of food science and technology-mysore 2004; 1;41(5): 586-90.

[81]   Grollier C, Debien C, Dornier M, Reynes M. Prominent characteristics and possible uses of the tamarind. Fruits 1998; 53(4): 271.

[82]   Jayaweera DM. Medicinal plants (Indigenous and exotic) used in Ceylon. Colombo: National Science Council of Sri Lanka 1981-1982.

[83]   De Caluwé E, Halamová K, Van Damme P. Baobab (*Adansonia digitata* L.): a review of traditional uses, phytochemistry and pharmacology. ACS Symposium Series 2010; 23(1).

[84]   Manohar B, Ramakrishna P, Udayasankar K. Some physical properties of tamarind (*Tamarindus indica* L.) juice concentrates. J Food Eng 1991; 13(4): 241-58.
[http://dx.doi.org/10.1016/0260-8774(91)90045-T]

[85]   Kiranmai E, Uma M, Vimala B. Squash from tamarind pulp by blending with mango pulp. Agric Update 12(TECHSEAR-6): 1660-5.

[86]   Kiranmai E, Uma M, Vimala B. Preparation of Tamarind Jam Blended with Mango. Int J Curr Microbiol Appl Sci (6): 12.
[http://dx.doi.org/10.20546/ijcmas.2017.612.392]

[87]   Adeola AA, Aworh CO. Development and sensory evaluation of an improved beverage from Nigeria's tamarind (*Tamarindus indica* L.) fruit. Afr J Food Agric Nutr Dev 2010; 10(9).
[http://dx.doi.org/10.4314/ajfand.v10i9.62888]

[88]   Adeola AA, Aworh OC. Effects of sodium benzoate on storage stability of previously improved beverage from tamarind (*Tamarindus indica* L.). Food Sci Nutr 2014; 2(1): 17-27.
[http://dx.doi.org/10.1002/fsn3.78] [PMID: 24804061]

[89]   Kaur G, Nagpal A, Kaur B. Tamarind, date of India, Science Tech Entrepreneur. National Science and Technology Entrepreneurship Development Board (2006), New Delhi 2006.

[90]   Rao YS, George CK. Tamarind – ideal for rainfed area, The Hindu, India. 1996.

[91]   Anon. Agmark Grade Specifications for Spices. 1996.

CHAPTER 3

An Overview of The Tamarind (*Tamarindus indica* L.) Fruit: A Potential source of Nutritional and Health Promoting Phytoconstituents

F. Lucy Oyetayo[1,*] and **I. Adebayo Odeniyi**[1]

Department of Biochemistry, Ekiti State University, Ado-Ekiti, Ekiti State, Nigeria

Abstract: The Tamarind fruit is an arboreal fruit of the Tamarind plant (*Tamarindus indica*), an unconventional fruiting tree that grows mostly in the wild. The fruit contains phytoconstituents with important food and therapeutic applications. The fruit extract has been shown to possess antimicrobial and health-promoting activities such as antioxidative, antidiabetic, hepatoprotective, and hypolipidemic properties. It is an important flavoring agent in food and beverage processing due to the aroma of its flavor constituents. The fruit is a potential source of readily available, affordable, natural nutritive, and medicinal components that can be exploited as a health-promoting food for the developing world.

Keywords: Antioxidative, Antidiabetic, Antinutrients, Hepatoprotective, Hypolipidemic, Medicinal, Nutritional, Phytoconstituents, Tamarind, Unconventional.

INTRODUCTION

The Tamarind plant (*Tamarindus indica*) is a fruit-bearing tree of the family Leguminosae, which bears one of the unconventional fruits found almost throughout the tropics and subtropics [1]. The tree grows in the wild though cultivated to a limited extent in Nigeria [2]. The most useful part of the plant; the fruit made up of the pulp and seed; is edible but underutilized. It possesses various nutritional and medicinal benefits [3] but the seeds have been reported to be gaining importance as an alternative protein source [4]. Typical Tamarind fruit contains about 55% pulp, 34% seeds, 11% shell, fibers [5], and other phytoconstituents with important food and therapeutic applications. It is a rich source of micro and macronutrients such as vitamins B and C which have important immune functions, nutritive mineral elements: calcium, phosphorus,

* **Corresponding author F. Lucy Oyetayo**: Department of Biochemistry, Ekiti State University, Ado-Ekiti, Ekiti State, Nigeria; Tel: +2348 060163 025; E-mail:ovounad@yahoo.com

Atta-ur-Rahman, M. Iqbal Choudhary & Sammer Yousuf (Eds.)

copper, and zinc [6] which serve as cofactors to various enzymes in physiology, and antinutrients: such as tannins, phenols, flavonoids and phytic acids which possess numerous medicinal values such as antimicrobial and health-promoting activities: antioxidative, antidiabetic, hepatoprotective and hypolipidemic properties. The tamarind seed oil contains high proportions of unsaturated fatty acids which makes it important in the control of cardiovascular disorders. Consumption of vegetables containing low n-6/n-3 fatty acids is highly associated with the reduction in the risk of developing various chronic diseases such as coronary heart disease [7]. It is an important flavoring agent in food and beverage processing with several industrial and commercial applications [4].

The incidence of malnutrition resulting from the intake of nutritionally deficient diets is a universal Public health problem especially in the rural areas of the developing world. It affects all geographies and all age groups leading to susceptibility and severity of infections [8].

The tamarind fruit, an underutilized edible fruit, is a potential source of readily available natural phytoconstituents especially being inexpensive, could help alleviate malnutrition which is widespread in the developing world where it could be exploited as a medicinal food.

BOTANICAL DESCRIPTION AND HISTORICAL CULTIVATION

The genus *Tamarindus* is a monotypic genus containing the sole species *T. indica* and belongs to the sub-family Caesalpinioideae of the family Fabaceae (Leguminosae) [9]. Tamarind is a large, evergreen tree, up to 24 m in height and 7 m in girth. A full-grown tamarind tree is reported to yield about 180–225 kg of fruits per season [10]. The tree grows in the tropical regions of the world [11] though it has become naturalized in many places particularly including Central African countries, and 36 other countries including India and Thailand where it was introduced [3]. However, tamarind is grown as a major plantation only in a few countries such as India and Thailand.

Tamarind fruits begin to ripen during the months of February-March. The fruits are allowed to ripen on the tree until the outer shell is dry and could be easily separated from the pulp without adherence [12]. The outermost covering is fragile and easily separable. The fruit contains 3-12 seeds, which are irregularly shaped, flattened, or rhomboid. The seeds are very hard, shiny, reddish, or purplish brown, enveloped by a tough leathery membrane, the so-called endocarp. Outside the endocarp is the light brownish-red, sweetish, acidic edible pulp traversed by tough ligneous fibers. The seed consists of the seed coat or testa (20-30%) and the kernel or endosperm (70-75%) [10].

CHEMICAL AND NUTRITIONAL COMPOSITION OF TAMARIND FRUIT

The most valuable and commonly used part of the Tamarind plant is the fruit which yields an acidic pulp [13] due to the content of tartaric acid (8-18%) present in the fruit. It is the dominant acid present in the tamarind fruit pulp which gives it an acidic taste although malic, succinic, and citric acids are also present. The whole seeds contain protein, fat, sugars, and carbohydrates. Compared to the pulp, tamarind seed is more abundant in protein (13–20%) and oil (4.5–16.2%). Relatively inexpensive sources of protein have been investigated by many researchers. Alternatives to expensive meat and meat products must be dietary staples affordable to high percentages of the population and readily available in abundant quantities [14]. Amino acid profiles of tamarind reveal that the proteins contain fairly balanced essential amino acid levels. *In vitro* protein digestibility of tamarind is 71.6% which is comparable to the levels reported for Soya beans [15]. The seed coat is rich in fiber (20%).

The major volatile constituents of tamarind pulp include furan derivatives (44.4%) and carboxylic acids (38.2%), which include furfural (38.2%), and phenylacetaldehyde (7.5%) [16]. The most abundant volatile constituent of tamarind is 2-acetyl-furan, coupled with traces of furfural and 5-methylfurfural, which form the total aroma of the tamarind fruit pulp. Among the fatty acids, linoleic, oleic, and palmitic acids are the major constituents. Linoleic acid, present in tamarind seed oil, is one of the most important polyunsaturated acids in human foods. A large body of literature supports the beneficial effects of polyunsaturated acids in health and disease [17].

Dehusked tamarind seeds are a source of pectin, (2-3.5%) the jelly-forming constituent of many fruits, vegetables, and seeds. The fruit also contains reducing sugars (25-45%) and cellulose. Besides being a rich source of sugars tamarind pulp is an excellent source of B-vitamins: riboflavin thiamin and niacin but poor in vitamins A and C [18]. Both pulp and seeds of the fruit are good sources of potassium, calcium, phosphorous, sodium, zinc and iron [19]. The anthocyanin pigment, called chrysanthemin is responsible for the color of the pulp in case of red variety of tamarind and the brown color of the pulp of brown variety is due to leucocyanidin [11].

ANTI-NUTRIENT COMPOSITION OF TAMARIND

Food legumes are important sources of dietary proteins in developing countries, but their acceptability and utilization have been limited due to the presence of relatively high concentrations of certain anti-nutritional factors [20]. In addition to its nutritive and medicinal components, the tamarind fruit is also a source of diverse forms of naturally occurring antinutritional factors including tannins, trypsin inhibitor (10.8), phytic acid and hydrogen cyanide [3]. Antinutrients act to reduce nutrient utilization and hence induce a deficiency state in an otherwise balanced diet [21]. Trypsin inhibitor activity in the fruit is higher in the pulp than the seed and it exhibits low inhibitory activity. The seed also contains 47 mg/100g of phytic acid, which has minimal effect on its nutritive value [22]. Phytic acid decreases the bioavailability of certain minerals and may interfere with the utilization of proteins due to the formation of phytate-protein and phytate-mineral complexes [20] and also inhibits the digestive enzymes Phytate could, however, be substantially eliminated by processing methods such as soaking and autoclaving. The presence of tannins and other antinutrients in the whole seed makes it unsuitable for direct human consumption without processing. Therefore, the testa has to be separated from the kernels by boiling, soaking, or roasting [21]. Otherwise, side effects such as depression, constipation, and gastrointestinal disorders may result from its consumption.

Tamarind seeds contain 2.8 mg/100g cyanogens, which is too low to cause any concern since cooking is known to reduce cyanogen content significantly, although it is a potent respiratory chain inhibitor with fatal consequences at high concentrations [23]. However, antinutrients possess certain health benefits. For instance, Phytate can influence the functional and nutritional properties of food, depending on its concentration. It also has the potential ability to lower blood glucose, reduce cholesterol and triacylglycerols, reduce risk of cancer through its absorption of divalent and multivalent minerals which cancerous cells require for growth [22]. Other beneficial effects of antinutrients include their hypolipidemic, antidiabetic and antioxidative properties.

FOOD USES OF TAMARIND

Due to its pleasant acidic taste and rich aroma, the pulp is widely used for domestic and industrial purposes [24]. The pulp is used as a seasoning, to flavor confections, curries, and sauces and as a substitute for chemical acidulants in the preparation of certain beverages. Tamarind pulp can be processed into several products including tamarind juice, concentrate, powder, pickles and paste [5]

The seeds, a by-product of the pulp industry, are usually wasted [4] hence, constituting a source of contamination and an environmental pollutant due to their content of compounds that can limit their direct use in soil or feed application [25]. However, instead of constituting health hazards, they could be ground to make a palatable livestock feed after processing.

Tamarind seed is also the raw material used in the manufacture of polysaccharide (jellose), adhesive, and tannin. Pectin with carbohydrate character and gelly forming properties, named 'jellose' has been recommended for use as a stabilizer in ice cream, mayonnaise and cheese, and as an ingredient or agent in several pharmaceutical products [4]. Flour from the seed may be made into cake and bread. Roasted seeds are claimed to be superior to groundnuts in flavor.

The major industrial product of tamarind seed is the tamarind kernel powder (TKP) which is an important sizing material used in the textile, paper, and jute industries.

MEDICINAL USES OF THE TAMARIND FRUIT

The fruit of the Tamarind plant possesses some medicinal properties such as digestive, carminative, laxative, and expectorant. The pulp has been found to possess hypolipidemic activity [26]. Intake of the fruit delays the progression of fluorosis in humans by enhancing the urinary excretion of fluorine [24]. In traditional practice, the pulp is applied on inflammations and also used in a gargle for sore throat. The pulp is said to aid the restoration of sensation in cases of paralysis [2].

It as an anthelminthic, antimicrobial, antiseptic, antiviral, sunscreen agent. The tamarind fruit has commonly been used throughout Southeast Asia as a poultice applied to the foreheads of fever sufferers [5].

Purified xyloglucan from tamarind has been used for conjunctiva cell adhesion and corneal wound healing in eye surgery.

Antioxidant Activities of Tamarind Fruit

There is increasing interest in the protective biological roles of natural antioxidants confined in dietary vegetation that are candidates for the deterrence of oxidative damage. Some of these antioxidants are polyphenol compounds that are found in all plant parts [26].

Several reports on the antioxidant activity of tamarind indicate that fruits have a high antioxidant capacity that can be considered beneficial to human health [27].

Antioxidant nutrients must be constantly replenished through diet or by dietary supplementation [28]. Four anti-oxidative compounds isolated and identified from the seed coat include; phenolic antioxidants, such as 2-hydroxy-3', 4'-dihydroxyacetophenone, methyl 3,4-dihydroxybenzoate, 3,4-dihydroxyphenyl acetate, and epicatechin [29]. Antioxidants may be used to increase the shelf life of food products and to improve the stability of lipids and lipid-containing foods by preventing loss of sensory and nutritional quality and lipid peroxidation. Raw and dry heated tamarind seed coats exhibited good antioxidant activities against the linoleic acid emulsion system compared to the synthetic antioxidant, butylated-hydroxy-anisole [30].

Sudjaroen *et al* [31] described the antioxidant activity of tamarind pericarp extract and reported the presence of mainly polymeric tannins and oligomeric procyanidins. Ethanol and ethyl acetate extracts of tamarind seed coats have been shown to exhibit anti-oxidative activity [32]. This suggests that a tamarind seed coat, a by-product of the tamarind gum industry, may serve as a potential source of low-cost antioxidants.

Antimicrobial Properties of the Tamarind Fruit

The fruits of tamarind are reported to have antifungal and antibacterial properties [11]. It is also reported to be a potent fungicidal agent to cultures of *Aspergillus niger* and *Candida albicans*. Extracts from tamarind fruit pulp have also shown molluscicidal activity against *Bulinus trancatus* snails. The antimicrobial activity of the tamarind fruit has been attributed to lupeol, a pharmacologically active triterpene [11].

Anti-Inflammatory Activities of Tamarind Fruit

Proteinase inhibitors with regulatory and defensive roles are widely distributed among bacteria, animals, and plants. They act as storage proteins. Among the various groups of proteinase inhibitors, serine proteinase inhibitors are the best studied and have been isolated from various leguminous seeds. A serine proteinase inhibitor, providing high activity against Human neutrophil elastase was detected, isolated, and purified from tamarind seeds [33]. Polyphenols and flavonoid content of *T. indica* have also been shown to possess anti-inflammatory properties [34].

Anticancer Activities of Tamarind Fruit

Cancer, a major life-threatening non-communicable disease in the world today, is a state of uncontrolled proliferation of cells linked to oxidative stress. However, secondary metabolites such as polyphenolic compounds such as tannins synthesized by plants have been found to possess powerful antioxidant properties protecting the human body from free radical damage [35]. Epidemiological data have indicated the beneficial effects of antioxidants in the prevention of cancer, cardiovascular and neurodegenerative disorders associated with aging [36]. *Tamarind indica* seed extract polyphenolics, based on their antioxidant properties, have been shown to improve chemical-induced acute nephrotoxicity and renal cell carcinoma in experimental trials. These polyphenols possess cancer-related signal pathway blockage effect and antioxidant enzyme induction properties [37].

CONCLUSION AND RECOMMENDATIONS

Tamarind is a versatile fruit with potentials as a source of nutritious and health benefiting phytoconstituents which possess certain industrial and commercial applications. Because of the overall nutrient and chemical composition, the fruit may be recommended as an inexpensive potential protein source, which can be exploited to alleviate malnutrition problems in the developing parts of the world.

Also, efforts should be geared towards genetic manipulation of the plant to yield nutrient-dense and medicinally beneficial phytoconstituents containing varieties of the plant fruit. Furthermore, popularization of the plant to promote large scale cultivation and possibly domestication should be encouraged. Isolation and characterization of various functional constituents of the fruit to elucidate their potential pharmacological activities are required.

CONSENT FOR PUBLICATION

Not applicable.

CONFLICT OF INTEREST

The authors confirm that there is no conflict of interest.

ACKNOWLEDGEMENTS

Declared none.

REFERENCES

[1]   Singh D, Wangchu L, Moond SK. Possessed products of tamarind. Nat Prod Rad 2007; 6(4): 315-21.

[2]   Mohammed D. Tamarind (Tamarindus indicus L) Fruit of Potential Value But Underutilized in Nigeria. International Journal of Innovative Food. Nutrition &Sustainable Agriculture 2019; 7(1): 1-10.

[3]   Kumar CS, Bhattacharya S. Tamarind seed: properties, processing and utilization. Crit Rev Food Sci Nutr 2008; 48(1): 1-20.
[PMID: 18274963]

[4]   El-Siddig K, Gunasena HM, Prasa BA. Tamarind-*Tamarindus indica* L. Fruits for the future 1. UK: Southampton Centre for Underutilized Crops Southampton 2006.

[5]   De Caluwe E, Halamov K, Van Damme P. Tamarind (Tamarindus indica L): A review of traditional uses, phytochemistry and pharmacology. HR Juliani, Ed. African natural plant products: discoveries and challenges in quality control. American chemical society, ACS Symposium Series 1021. Washington DC, US 2010; pp. 85-110.

[6]   Okello J, Okullo JBL, Eilu G, Nyeko P, Obua J. Mineral composition of *Tamarindus indica* LINN (tamarind) pulp and seeds from different agro-ecological zones of Uganda. Food Sci Nutr 2017; 5(5): 959-66.
[http://dx.doi.org/10.1002/fsn3.490] [PMID: 28948013]

[7]   Simopoulos AP. Omega-3 fatty acids and antioxidants in edible wild plants. Biol Res 2004; 37(2): 263-77.
[PMID: 15455656]

[8]   Report GN. Shining a light to spur action on nutrition. north Quary House Temple Back Bristol BS1 6FL,Bristal, UK 1-161: Development Initiatives Poverty Res Ltd 2018.

[9]   Kirtikar KR, Basu BD. Indian Medicinal Plants. 3rd. 1987; 2: pp. 887-91.

[10]   FAO. Tropical Food Plants, FAO Food and Nutrition. A resource book for Promoting Fatty acid and sterol composition of Malagasy tamarind kernels 1998.

[11]   Shaikh Z, Mujahid M, Bagga P, *et al.* Medicinal uses & pharmacological activity of *Tamarindus indica* World. J Pharm Sci 2017; 5(2): 121-33.http://www.wjpsonline.org/

[12]   Shankaracharya NB. Tamarind-Chemistry, Technology and Uses-A Critical Appraisal. J Food Sci Technol 1998; 35(3): 193-208.

[13]   Jyothirmayi T, Rao GN, Rao DG. Studies on instant raw tamarind chutney powder. J Fd Serv 2006; 17(3): 119-23.

[14]   Oyetayo FL, Oyetayo VO. Assessment of nutritional quality of wild and cultivated *Pleurotus sajor-caju.* J Med Food 2009; 12(5): 1149-53.
[PMID: 19857082]

[15]   Andrade VR, Leonel VP, Villela SDJ, *et al.* Soybean in different forms of processing in the feeding of crossbred cows on brachiaria grass pastures R. Bras Zootech 2015; 44(2): 37-43.

[16]   Wong KL, Tan CP, Chow CH, *et al.* Volatile constituents of the fruit of *Tamarindus indica* L. Ess Oil Research 1998; 10(2): 219-21.

[17]   Leng S, Winter T, Aukema HM. Dietary ALA, EPA and DHA have distinct effects on oxylipin profiles in female and male rat kidney, liver and serum. J Nutr Biochem 2018; 57: 228-37.
[PMID: 29778015]

[18]   Caluwé e de, Halamová K, Van damme P, *et al.* Tamarind (*Tamarindus indica*) Subtropical Fruits Westport, CT, 375: AVI Publishing 2009.

[19]   Popova A, Mihaylova D. Antinutrients in plant-based foods: a review. Open Biotechnol J 2019; 13: 68-76.

[20]   Oyetayo FL, Ibitoye MF. Phytochemical and nutrient/antinutrient interactions in cherry tomato (Lycopersicon esculentum) fruits. Nutr Health 2012; 21(3): 187-92.
[PMID: 23533206]

[21]   Samtiya M, Aluko RE, Dhewa T. Plant food anti-nutritional factors and their reduction strategies: an overview Fd processing & Nutr 6 2020; 1-14.

[22]   Ishola MM, Agbaji EB, Agbaji AS. A chemical study on *Tamarindus indica* (Tsamiya) fruits grown in Nig. J Sci Food Agric 1990; 51(1): 141-3.

[23]   Botham KM, Mayes PA. Respiratory Chain and Oxidative Phosphorylation in Harper's Illustrated Biochemistry Murray R.K Eds. Lange Medical Books. 27th edn., New York, San Fransisco , Libson, London: McGraw-Hill Medical Publishing Division 2006.Pp100-107

[24]   Obulesu M, Bhattacharya S. Color Changes of *Tamarindus indica* L. pulp during fruit development, ripening and storage. Int J Food Prop 2011; 14(3): 538-49.

[25]   Costa S G A, Alves R C, Vinha AF, *et al.* Nutritional Chemical and antioxidant/pro-oxidant profile of silverskin, a coffee roasting by-product Fd Chem267 2018; 28-35.

[26]   Martinello F, Soares SM, Franco JJ, *et al.* Hypolipemic and antioxidant activities from *Tamarindus indica* L. pulp fruit extract in hypercholesterolemic hamsters. Food Chem Toxicol 2006; 44(6): 810-8.
[PMID: 16330140]

[27]   Khandare A, Rasaputra K, Meshram I, Rao S. Effects of smoking, use of aluminium utensils, and tamarind consumption on fluorosis in a fluorotic village of Andhra Pradesh, India, Research Report. Fluoride 2010; 43(2): 128-33. [The International Society for Fluoride Research Inc].

[28]   Oyetayo FL, Ojo OA. *Dennetia tripetala* seeds inhibit ferrous sulphate-induced oxidative stress in rat tissue *in vitro*. Oxid Antioxid Med Sci 2017; 6(2): 35-9.
       [http://dx.doi.org/10.5455/oams.110417.or.104]

[29]   Tsuda T, Watanable M, Ohshima K, Yamanato A, Kawakishi S, Osawa T. Antioxidative components isolated from the seed of tamarind (*Tamarindus indica* L.) Journal of Agric and Fd chem 1994; 42: 1674-2671.

[30]   Siddhuraju P. Antioxidant activity of polyphenolic compounds extracted from defatted raw and dry heated *Tamarindus indica* seed coat. LWT Fd Sci and Tech 2007; 40: 982-90.

[31]   Sudjaroen Y, Haubner R, Würtele G, *et al.* Isolation and structure elucidation of phenolic antioxidants from Tamarind (*Tamarindus indica* L.) seeds and pericarp. Food Chem Toxicol 2005; 43(11): 1673-82.
       [PMID: 16000233]

[32]   Osawa T, Tsuda T, Watanabe M, Hshima K, Yamamoto A. Antioxidative components isolated from the seeds of tamarind (*Tamarindus indica* L.). J Agric Food Chem 1994; 42(12): 2671-4.

[33]   Fook JM, Macedo LL, Moura GE, *et al.* A serine proteinase inhibitor isolated from *Tamarindus indica* seeds and its effects on the release of human neutrophil elastase. Life Sci 2005; 76(25): 2881-91.
       [PMID: 15820500]

[34]   Samuelsson G, Bohlin L. Drugs of Natural Origin: A Treatise of Pharmacognosy. CRC Press Inc; Halliwell (1996) Antioxidants in health and disease. Annu Rev Nutr 2017; 16: 39-50.

[35]   Halliwell B. Antioxidants in human health and disease. Annu Rev Nutr 1996; 16: 33-50.
       [PMID: 8839918]

[36]   Burda S, Oleszek W. Antioxidant and antiradical activities of flavonoids. J Agric Food Chem 2001; 49(6): 2774-9.
       [PMID: 11409965]

[37]   Saha S, Pal D, Kumar S. Hydroxyacetamide Derivatives: Cytotoxicity genotoxicity, antioxidative and metal chelating studies. Indian J Exp Biol 2017; 55(12): 831-7.

CHAPTER 4

The Clinical Overview of Turmeric, Turmeric-based Medicines, and Turmeric Isolates

Elin Y. Sukandar and **Dhyan K. Ayuningtyas**

Department of Pharmacology and Clinical Pharmacy, School of Pharmacy, Bandung Institute of Technology, Bandung, Indonesia

Abstract: Turmeric (*Curcuma longa* Linn), which belongs to the Zingiberaceae family, is one of the most well-known and thoroughly studied medicinal plants, and is also one of the few medicinal plants that have been scientifically proven to be beneficial to human health. The most frequently used part of turmeric is the rhizome, for which several studies have reported to contain high levels of beneficial essential oils and numerous chemical constituents. One of the most well-studied chemical constituents of turmeric is curcumin, which has exhibited the ability to target multiple signaling pathways while also demonstrating certain pharmacological activities at the cellular level in preclinical studies. Advancing these preclinical studies, numerous clinical studies on various diseases involving turmeric-based medication have been conducted, including dyspepsia, irritable bowel syndrome, peptic ulcer, and cancer lesions, among various other diseases. We report an extensive examination of the clinical aspect of turmeric and turmeric-based medication, including its isolates. This review provides a comprehensive overview of the state-of-the-art clinical studies involving turmeric and its effects on various diseases.

Keywords: Curcumin, *Curcuma longa*, Clinical Studies, Formulation, Herbal Medicine, Turmeric, Zingiberaceae.

INTRODUCTION

Sources of traditional medicine generally include other materials aside from plants, such as honey, parts of animals, and any natural organic or inorganic, active ingredients. However, the main ingredients of herbal medicine are derived from plants and plant materials. According to the World Health Organization (WHO), herbal medicines may be available in the form of herbs, herbal materials, herbal preparations, and finished herbal products, which are labeled medicinal products with an active ingredient, part of plants, or a combination of various plants.

---

* **Corresponding author Elin Y. Sukandar:** Pharmacy, School of Pharmacy Bandung Institute of Technology Indonesia; Tel: +628990356323, +6281320552054; E-mail: eyulinah@gmail.com

Atta-ur-Rahman, M. Iqbal Choudhary & Sammer Yousuf (Eds.)

In some countries, herbal medicines may also contain, by tradition, natural organic or inorganic active ingredients that are not of plant origin, such as animal and mineral materials. Even though regulations and definitions of herbal medicine vary between countries, there is the consensus that all preparations supplemented with chemically defined active substances, including synthetic compound and/or isolated constituents from herbal materials, are not considered as herbal medicine [1, 2].

Herbal products have become an important and inseparable part of the modern healthcare system. Nevertheless, embracing the use of herbal medicine in healthcare is not without obstacles, and several issues need to be addressed, such as safety, regulation, and product standardization (quality control), as well as financial and ethical aspects [3]. Preclinical studies of herbal medicine do not always provide satisfactory evidence of the efficacy and safety of herbal medicine, and clinical trials are still essential for the development of herbal medicine.

Unlike conventional medicine, of which there is a near-unanimous agreement, many countries have different regulations regarding clinical trials of herbal medicine. Developed countries, such as the US, classify herbal products as supplements, hence the conventional phases of clinical trials cannot be applied for these products [4]. On the other hand, countries like Indonesia implement the same regulations of clinical trials of conventional medicine as for traditional medicine [5]. The differences in regulations between countries cause difficulties in head-to-head comparisons in evaluating the clinical efficacy of herbal medicine. To prevent discrepancies in the clinical trial evaluation of herbal medicine, WHO released in 2013 an operational guideline outlining the information needed to support clinical trials of herbal products [6]. This operational guideline contains chemistry manufacturing control (standardization) for herbal products, non-clinical considerations, clinical considerations, and ethical considerations in clinical trials for herbal products.

One of the most well-known and thoroughly studied medicinal plants in clinical trials is turmeric (*Curcuma longa* L.). This plant is widely cultivated in tropical areas of Asia and Central America, but its use is different between these areas. Turmeric is a minor spice in the West, but it is a major spice in the East with numerous applications such as in coloring (dye), as food preservatives, cosmetics, and herbal remedies [7, 8]. Although the utilization of turmeric differs in Eastern and Western cultures, the use of turmeric as herbal medicine is quite popular around the world.

The most frequently used part of turmeric is the rhizome, which several studies have reported to have a high content of beneficial essential oils and numerous chemical constituents [9]. Some of these chemical constituents have been successfully isolated from turmeric, but the most distinct and extensively studied from various aspects, including in clinical trials, is curcumin.

Turmeric has demonstrated various pharmacological effects in both preclinical and clinical studies. Numerous clinical studies investigating the efficacy of turmeric or turmeric-based medication on various diseases have been conducted. These diseases include cancer, cardiovascular disease, arthritis, uveitis, ulcerative proctitis, Crohn's disease, ulcerative colitis, irritable bowel disease, tropical pancreatitis, peptic ulcer, gastric ulcer, idiopathic orbital inflammatory pseudotumor, oral lichen planus, gastric inflammation, vitiligo, psoriasis, acute coronary syndrome, atherosclerosis, diabetes, diabetic nephropathy, diabetic microangiopathy, lupus nephritis, renal conditions, acquired immunodeficiency syndrome, β-thalassemia, biliary dyskinesia, cholecystitis, and chronic bacterial prostatitis [10]. Some of these clinical studies showed promising results and have continued to advanced phases, while others stopped at an early phase. Both are included in this chapter as considerations on the development of turmeric in the near future.

Although turmeric and its isolates have been proven beneficial in numerous preclinical studies, the poor bioavailability associated with poor absorption, rapid metabolism, and rapid elimination has hindered the utilization of turmeric in clinical settings [11, 12]. Several formulations have been developed and tested to improve its bioavailability, hence the various clinical studies detailed in this chapter used different formulations. Well-designed clinical trials supported by appropriate formulation and administration are crucial to ensure that the benefits of turmeric-based medication can be reproduced in diverse settings. This chapter provides comprehensive prevailing knowledge of the clinical aspect of turmeric and turmeric-based medications, including its isolates, even though isolates are not classified as herbal medicine.

CLINICAL STUDIES

The discussion of clinical studies in this chapter is divided into two segments, namely the clinical studies of turmeric or turmeric-based medication, and clinical studies of the chemical constituents of turmeric, including turmeric isolates, which mainly focuses on curcumin. Several clinical studies investigated the use of turmeric or turmeric-based medication as a single agent, while others investigated the use of turmeric in combination with other traditional medicine. This chapter does not differentiate between the use of turmeric as a single agent or in combination with other herbal medicines, and both uses are explored in detail. The number of clinical studies of turmeric without any further processing is quite limited, although there is some explanation in the clinical study of turmeric isolates. However, this chapter focuses mainly on turmeric, and only trending clinical studies on turmeric isolates are reviewed.

Clinical Studies of Turmeric and Turmeric-based Medicine

Clinical studies of turmeric medication in this chapter covers the use of turmeric and turmeric-based medicine. The discussion of turmeric-based medication in this chapter includes turmeric extract, with or without fractioning, and turmeric formulations that only affect turmeric delivery or the pharmacokinetics of turmeric without altering its pharmacodynamics profile.

Turmeric has been tested on various diseases on humans. It is predicted to be able to assist in the management of oxidative and inflammatory conditions in general, such as the management of soreness and pain in patients with arthritis. Turmeric also helps in the management of metabolic diseases, although this use is not as popular as its use in the treatment of inflammatory-related conditions. It also helped in the treatment of various cancers with multiple mechanisms. Furthermore, a relatively low dosage of turmeric may promote health conditions in healthy subjects [13].

Arthritis

Madhu *et al.* evaluated the benefit of turmeric in patients with knee osteoarthritis. The study was a randomized controlled study at a university hospital in Bangkok, Thailand. In this study, 107 patients with primary knee osteoarthritis (OA) with a pain score of more than 5 were randomized to receive either ibuprofen 800 mg per day or turmeric extracts 2 g per day for 6 weeks. After 6 weeks, improvements in pain on level walking, pain on climbing stairs, and knee functions assessed by the time spent on a 100-meter walk and going up and down a flight of stairs were measured. Compared to the baseline, the efficacy parameters at weeks 2, 4, and 6 were significantly improved in both the groups. There was no difference in the parameters between the patients receiving ibuprofen and those receiving turmeric extracts, except for pain on climbing stairs ($p = 0.016$) [14].

Another study on arthritis was performed by Gupta *et al.* using the investigational product NR-INF-02, which was a polysaccharide-rich turmeric extract, hence categorized as a turmeric product in this section. The study was a randomized, single-blind, placebo-controlled trial. A total of 120 patients (37 males and 83 females) with primary knee OA received either placebo (400 mg twice daily), NR-INF-02 (500 mg twice daily), glucosamine sulfate (GS) (750 mg twice daily), or a combination of NR-INF-02 and GS, for 42 days. The primary efficacy outcomes measured were the decrease in the severity of pain symptom and function of the affected knee, determined after 42 days. The outcomes were assessed using the Visual Analog Scale (VAS) for pain symptom and Western Ontario and McMaster Universities Osteoarthritis Index (WOMAC) scale for knee function. The clinical examination of the affected joint was also measured using a Clinician Global Impression Change (CGIC) scale. Post-treatment scores using VAS, WOMAC, and CGIC assessed on day 21 and 42 showed significant improvement ($P < 0.05$) compared to placebo. In addition, the NR-INF-02 treated group showed a significant decrease ($P < 0.01$) in the needs of using rescue medication compared to placebo in this study [15].

In addition, Henrotin *et al.* investigated the bio-optimized *Curcuma longa* extract (BCL) on the management of knee osteoarthritis. This study was a prospective, randomized, 3-month, double-blind, multicenter, three-group, placebo-controlled trial. A total of 150 patients were randomized for treatment with low dose BCL 2 × 2 capsules/day, high dose BCL 2 × 3 capsules/day, or placebo, for 3 months. Each capsule contained 46.67 mg of turmeric rhizome extract. The Patient Global Assessment of Disease Activity (PGADA) measure and serum sColl2-1, a biomarker of cartilage degradation, were evaluated as the primary endpoints, while VAS, Knee injury, and the Osteoarthritis Outcome Score (KOOS), along with paracetamol/non-steroidal anti-inflammatory drug (NSAID) consumption, were used as secondary endpoints. Both low and high doses of BCL decreased PGAD better than placebo, and there was a transient increase of sColl2-1 in both the low dose BCL and placebo groups, but the differences were statistically insignificant for both of these parameters. The VAS analysis showed that both high and low doses of BCL significantly decreased knee pain ($P < 0.001$). The KOOS global score showed improvement over time in all groups ($P < 0.001$), but there were no differences for all groups, which implied that even the placebo group showed improvement without intervention after 3 months. There was a significant increase in adverse events (AE) related to the product in the high dose BCL group compared to the low dose BCL and placebo groups (37%, 21%, 13%, respectively, $P = 0.012$) [16].

A meta-analysis performed by Daily *et al.*, analyzed several randomized clinical trials of turmeric extracts and curcumin for the treatment or alleviating the symptoms of arthritis. The evaluated studies were obtained from 12 electronic databases, including PubMed, Embase, Cochrane Library, Korean databases, Chinese medical databases, and the Indian scientific database. As mentioned in the previous study, pain visual analog score (PVAS) and Western Ontario and McMaster Universities Osteoarthritis Index (WOMAC) were used as the primary outcome for arthritis. Only 8 studies met the selection criteria in this meta-analysis. Three studies reported a reduction of PVAS (mean difference: −2.04 [−2.85, −1.24]) with turmeric/curcumin compared to the placebo ($P < 0.00001$), while four studies showed a decrease in WOMAC with turmeric/curcumin treatment (mean difference: -15.36 $[-26.9, -3.77]$ compared to the placebo ($P < 0.01$). Unfortunately, the total number of RCTs included in the analysis, the relatively small sample size, and the methodological quality of the studies were still not sufficient to conclude the benefit of curcumin for arthritis [17].

Asthma

A randomized, double-blind, placebo-controlled, phase II clinical study was conducted by Manarin *et al.* to evaluate the efficacy of turmeric in addition to standard treatment for children and adolescents with persistent asthma. Patients were randomized to be given 30 mg/kg/day of *C. longa* for 6 months or placebo, on top of the standard therapy for asthma based on the severity of the disease. At the end of the treatment period, there was no difference in the frequency of symptoms and interference with normal activity between the turmeric and placebo groups [18].

Chemoprevention

One of the earliest clinical studies assessing the antimutagenic effect of turmeric on chronic smokers was performed by Polasa *et al.* This study was performed on 16 chronic smokers by administering 1.5 g/day of tablet preparations, each containing 750 mg of turmeric, for 30 days. Six non-smokers served as a control in this study. The results showed that giving turmeric significantly reduced the urinary excretion of mutagens in smokers, but had no significant effect on serum aspartate aminotransferase, alanine aminotransferase, blood glucose, creatinine, and lipid profiles [19]. This study was one of the early findings that indicated the benefits of turmeric as antimutagenic agents, and probably even as a chemoprevention agents, but the sample size was quite small.

Colorectal Cancer

A dose-escalation pilot study was performed by Sharma *et al.*, to evaluate the efficacy of a novel standardized Curcuma extract in proprietary capsule form at doses of 440–2200 mg/day towards colorectal cancer patients. Fifteen patients with advanced colorectal cancer refractory to standard chemotherapies were included in this study and received turmeric extract daily for up to 4 months. The activity of glutathione S-transferase and levels of a DNA adduct (M1G) formed by malondialdehyde were measured as efficacy parameters in this study. Patients who were taking 440 mg turmeric extract for 29 days showed a 59% decrease in lymphocytic glutathione S-transferase activity, but the same effect was not observed at the higher dose. Leukocytic M1G was not affected by the treatments, even at the highest dose [20]. This study showed highly variable results, but it is probably due to small sample sizes and the low bioavailability of turmeric constituents in the body.

Diabetes Mellitus

Sukandar *et al.*, evaluated the efficacy of turmeric extract in combination with garlic (*Allium sativum* L.) extract as an antidiabetic agent in comparison with glibenclamide. This was a double-blind, parallel, randomized control trial conducted in 14 weeks. Thirty-five patients were divided into two groups for 14 weeks of treatment and assessment. One group received a turmeric and garlic combination 3x2 capsules per day (each capsule containing 200 mg turmeric and 200 mg garlic extract), and the other group received 1 capsule of 5 mg glibenclamide per day. After 14 weeks of treatment, the group that received the extract combination showed a significant decrease in fasting blood glucose (192.76 *vs* 141.71 mg/dL), 2 hours post-prandial blood glucose (295.35 *vs* 204.35 mg/dL), and HbA1C (10.41 *vs* 8.09). The inter-group analysis showed $P > 0.05$ when compared to the glibenclamide group, implying the comparable effect of antidiabetic activity between turmeric-garlic combination and glibenclamide [21].

Another study by Wickenberg *et al.*, performed on healthy subjects assessed the effect of turmeric extract on postprandial plasma glucose and insulin. In this crossover trial, administering 6 g of curcumin capsules had no significant effect on the glucose response during a standard 75 g oral glucose tolerance test (OGTT) compared to the placebo group. However, this resulted in a significantly higher serum insulin response after 30 min ($P = 0.048$) and 60 min ($P = 0.033$), implying curcumin may affect insulin secretion in general [22].

Dyslipidemia

Another study was also performed by Sukandar *et al.* [23], to evaluate the antihyperglycemic and antihyperlipidemic effects of turmeric and garlic extract combination. Three doses of extract combination were evaluated in this study; 1.2, 1.6, and 2.4 g daily. The treatment was given for 14 weeks and assessed every 2 weeks. There were no placebo or reference drugs used as a comparison in this study, but the results showed no significant decrease in total cholesterol, LDL, and triglyceride levels compared to before the treatment of extract combination.

Sukandar *et al.* continued the previous clinical study, focusing on dyslipidemia patients without including those with diabetes mellitus condition. The study design was nearly identical to the previous study with the addition of a simvastatin (standard drug) group as a comparison. Thirty-nine subjects were included in this study; one group received 2.4 g of turmeric and garlic combination extract daily in two divided doses and another group received 5 mg simvastatin daily. The treatment was given for 12 weeks and assessed every 2 weeks. The results showed comparable results with simvastatin 5 mg in an overall lipid profile analysis. There were no adverse events related to the extract administration and there was a marked improvement in liver function at the end of the study in the turmeric-garlic group [24].

In addition, Qin *et al.* conducted a meta-analysis to assess the efficacy and safety of turmeric and curcumin in lowering blood lipids in patients with the risk of cardiovascular disease (CVD). The analysis included randomized controlled trials that assessed the effect of turmeric and curcumin on various parameters of blood lipid levels, including total cholesterol (TC), low-density lipoprotein cholesterol (LDL-C), high-density lipoprotein cholesterol (HDL-C), and triglycerides (TG). Only 7 studies met the selection criteria in this meta-analysis. Turmeric and curcumin significantly reduced serum LDL-C and TG levels ($P < 0.01$) compared to the control group, while serum HDL-C levels of the patients did not improve. In this meta-analysis, turmeric and curcumin showed a beneficial effect in protecting patients with the risk of cardiovascular disease through improving the LDL-C and TG levels, and appeared safe with no serious adverse events through all of the studies. However, the sample size was relatively small to draw a definite conclusion [25].

Human Gut Microbiota

Peterson *et al.* conducted a study to evaluate the effect of turmeric and curcumin dietary supplementation on human gut microbiota. The study was a double-blind, randomized, placebo-controlled pilot trial. The patients were randomized to receive either turmeric tablets with extract of piperine (Bioperine) (n = 6), curcumin with Bioperine tablets (n = 5), or placebo tablets (n = 3). The alteration in the gut microbiota was determined by 16S rDNA sequencing. The number of bacteria detected was 172-325 bacterial species. The results showed a highly personalized response to treatment; the turmeric and curcumin groups showed a 7% and 69% increase in detected bacterial species, respectively, while the placebo group showed a 15% reduction in detected species, post-treatment. This high variability in the results is to be expected due to the small sample size [26].

Lupus Nephritis

A study was performed by Khajehdehi *et al.* to evaluate the efficacy of turmeric extract in treating lupus nephritis. The study was a randomized and placebo-controlled study conducted at The Lupus Clinic of Hafez Hospital, Shiraz, Iran. A total of 24 patients with relapsing or refractory biopsy-proven lupus nephritis were included in this study and randomized into two groups, trial (n=12) and control (n=12) groups. Each patient in the trial group received 1 capsule containing 500 mg turmeric for 3 months, while the patients in the control group received capsules containing starch. After 3 months, a significant decrease in proteinuria was observed when comparing pre- (954.2 ± 836.6) and 1, 2, and 3 months supplementation values (448.8 ± 633.5, 235.9 ± 290.1, and 260.9 ± 106.2, respectively) in the trial group. Unfortunately, this study failed to show a significant effect ($P < 0.05$) when the trial group was compared to the placebo group [27].

Peptic Ulcer

The first study was performed by Van *et al.* [28], in which the healing effect of turmeric on the duodenal ulcer was evaluated. The study was a joint Vietnam-Sweden prospective, double-blind two-center study using 6 grams daily of turmeric tablets compared to the placebo. A total of 130 patients were included in this study; only patients having one duodenal ulcer with a minimum diameter of 5 mm verified by endoscopy and/or radiography for more than 4 days prior to the study were recruited. The results of this study showed that there was no significant difference between the turmeric group and placebo in ulcer healing rate. In contrast, there was an increase in side effects in the turmeric group compared to the placebo group (36% *vs* 20%), but this was deemed insignificant and may be related to ulcer disease itself [28].

A similar study was performed by Prucksunand *et al.*, on patients who had peptic ulcer symptoms. Forty-five patients were included in this study, but only 25 patients were confirmed to have ulcers located in the duodenal bulb and the angulus. Unlike the previous study, both gastric ulcers (GU) and duodenal ulcers (DU) were included in this study. Turmeric was given 3 g daily in five divided doses, one half to an hour before meals, at 16.00 hours and at bedtime continuously. The results showed that after 4 weeks of treatment, ulcers were absent in 48% (12 DU and GU 3) of patients. This number increased to 72% (DU 13 and GU 5) after 8 weeks of treatment and 76% after 12 weeks (DU 14 and GU 5). However, the results of this study are questionable since there was no placebo group for comparison. The previous study also showed that ulcers may be able to heal without medical aid, as can be seen in the placebo group of the first study [29].

Skin Inflammation

Asada *et al.*, investigated the potential for turmeric in the form of hot water extract to prevent skin inflammation. The study was a randomized, double-blind, placebo controlled trial for 8 weeks of intervention. In this study, a total of 47 healthy participants were given daily hot water extract of turmeric, with or without curcumin, or placebo. The turmeric administration significantly increased the water content of the face after 4-8 weeks of treatment compared to placebo. However, the addition of curcumin to the hot water extract of turmeric did not exhibit the same result. All groups failed to show a significant difference in trans-epidermal water loss and minimal erythema compared to the placebo [30]. Topical administration of turmeric with a proper formulation is predicted to be a better delivery system to maximize the effect of turmeric on the skin.

Vascular Function

Srinivasan *et al.* evaluated the effect of turmeric on arterial stiffness and endothelial dysfunction in patients with type 2 diabetes mellitus. The study was a randomized, double-blind, placebo-controlled study. A total of 136 patients were randomized to be given turmeric 400 mg thrice daily or placebo. Turmeric showed a significant reduction from baseline of carotid-femoral pulse wave velocity ($P = 0.002$), left brachial-ankle pulse wave velocity ($P = 0.001$), aortic augmentation pressure ($P = 0.007$), aortic augmentation index ($P = 0.007$), and aortic augmentation index at heart rate 75 ($P = 0.018$) compared with the placebo group. Turmeric significantly decreased the arterial stiffness compared to the placebo in type 2 diabetes mellitus patients after 3 months [31].

Clinical Studies of Turmeric Isolates

Of the many chemical constituents of turmeric, the curcuminoids are mainly responsible for its medicinal properties. One of the major characteristics of turmeric is the presence of curcumin (diferuloylmethane), an active constituent with numerous pharmacological properties. Other components of turmeric are demethoxycurcumin; bisdemethoxycurcumin; various volatile oils including turmerone, atlantone, and zingiberone; and minor components like sugars, proteins, and resins [32, 33]. The most extensively studied constituent is curcumin; hence this section will mainly focus on curcumin clinical studies.

Curcumin is available in various forms including capsules, tablets, ointments, energy drinks, soaps, and cosmetics [10]. Curcumin itself is known for its high tolerability and safety at high doses in humans. In a study involving gemcitabine-resistant patients with pancreatic cancer, the patients can tolerate 8 g oral curcumin daily in combination with gemcitabine-based chemotherapy [10, 15]. Although curcumin is well known for its multiple pharmacological properties in preclinical studies, curcumin is also infamous for its poor bioavailability in clinical studies. Numerous studies have revealed that curcumin has poor absorption, biodistribution, metabolism, and bioavailability. Some studies have shown that curcumin undergoes a rapid metabolism, largely in the intestinal mucosa and liver, and most of the substance passes through the gastrointestinal tract unchanged when consumed. Intestinal metabolism, specifically glucuronidation and sulfation of curcumin, may explain the poor systemic availability when curcumin is administered *via* the oral route, the most frequent administration route of curcumin. Various strategies were rendered to enhance the bioavailability of curcumin, from formulating nano-sized particles of curcumin, PLGA-encapsulated curcumin, liposomal encapsulation, encapsulation with cyclodextrin, and inhibiting hepatic and intestinal glucuronidation using piperine [12, 33, 34].

Alzheimer's Disease

One of the first studies conducted to evaluate the effect of curcumin on patients with a nervous-system related disease was performed by Baum *et al.* in patients with Alzheimer's disease (AD). The study was a randomized, placebo-controlled, double-blind, pilot clinical trial. A total of 34 patients who have had a progressive decline in memory and cognitive function for 6 months were randomized to receive either capsules of or powdered (4 g/1 g) curcumin once daily combined with 1 capsule (120 mg) of standardized ginkgo leaf extract, or placebo for 6 months. There was no difference in mini-mental state examination (MMSE) scores between the curcumin and placebo groups, but there was an increase in plasma Aβ40 levels [35].

In another study performed by Ringman *et al.*, turmeric was evaluated with the same study design as the previous study, but instead of 24 weeks (6 months), the study can be extended to 48 months as an open-label study. A total of 36 patients with AD were randomized to receive the placebo, 2 g/day curcumin, or 4 g/day curcumin. After completion of the study, no differences were observed in the MMSE score, Alzheimer's Disease Assessment Scale - Cognitive Subscale (ADAS-Cog), Neuropsychiatric Inventory (NPI), and the Alzheimer's Disease Cooperative Study - Activities of Daily Living (ADCS-ADL) scale. None were also observed in biomarker levels, including plasma Aβ1-40 and Aβ1-42, and cerebrospinal fluid levels of Aβ1-42, t-tau, p-tau181 and F2-isoprostanes between the turmeric and placebo groups [36]. The same result from a larger sample size (n = 96) was also observed in the study conducted by Rainey-Smith *et al*; after 12 months of study, there were no differences in clinical parameters between patients who received Biocurcumax™ (standardized extract of *C. longa* (88% curcuminoids and 7% volatile oil)) 1500 mg/day and placebo [37]. In non-demented patients, curcumin (n = 29) was found to improve memory and attention. It was suggested that symptom benefits are associated with decreases in amyloid and tau accumulation in the brain regions modulating mood and memory [38].

Beta-Thalassemia

A clinical study was conducted by Kalpravidh *et al*. to evaluate the efficacy of curcuminoid in improving the oxidative stress and antioxidant parameters in β-thalassemia/Hb E patients. In this study, a total of 21 β-thalassemia/Hb E patients (7 males and 14 females) were included. All patients were heterozygous for β0-thalassemia and Hb E, and had not received a blood transfusion, and 4 patients were splenectomized. The Hb concentrations were in the 60–80 g/L range. The patients in this study were recruited from the Division of Hematology, Department of Medicine, Faculty of Medicine Siriraj Hospital, Thailand. Two capsules of 250 mg curcuminoids were given daily to all patients for 12 months. The blood samples were collected every 2 months during treatment and 3 months following the completion of the treatments. The efficacy parameters were determined by measuring complete blood count, malonyldialdehyde (MDA), superoxide dismutase (SOD), glutathione peroxidase (GSH-Px), reduced glutathione (GSH) in red blood cells (RBC), and non-transferrin bound iron (NTBI) in serum. Increased oxidative stress in β-thalassemia/Hb E patients is shown by higher levels of MDA, SOD, GSH-Px in RBC, and serum NTBI, and lower levels of RBC GSH. As a control group, 26 healthy volunteers (9 males and 17 females) who had normal hemoglobin typing (Hb A and A2) were included. Curcumin was found to improve the patients' condition by decreasing MDA, RBC SOD, RBC GSH-Px, RBC GSH, and NTBI serum significantly ($P < 0.05$) after 6 months of treatment compared to the baseline. However, the effect was not maintained when the patients stopped taking curcumin. Although curcumin may have improved patients' conditions in this study, they are not comparable to those of healthy volunteers. There was no direct comparison to placebo or active comparators in this study [39].

Breast Cancer

An open-label phase 1 dose-escalation study for breast cancer was performed by Bayet-Robert *et al*. This study was conducted to evaluate the feasibility and tolerability of the combination of curcumin and docetaxel towards patients with advanced and metastatic breast cancer. Curcumin was administered orally from 500 mg/day and increased until a certain limited toxicity occurred, while docetaxel was administered as infusion at 100 mg/m^2 every three weeks for six cycles. Fourteen patients were included in this study, but only nine patients were evaluable; three patients refused to continue because of intolerance, one patient died after the first cycle and one patient had no clinical target. In all nine patients, no progressive disease was observed during treatment with a combination of curcumin and docetaxel. Eight patients (5 patients with partial response and 3 patients with stable disease) had measurable lesions based on the RECIST criteria.

The biological response showed up to a 50% decrease of tumor markers in 4 patients, but the authors did not disclose the complete results of tumor markers from all patients. The recommended dose from this study was 6000 mg/day for seven consecutive days, since higher doses resulted in intolerance for the patients [40].

Colorectal Cancer

Colorectal cancer is one of the most frequent diseases studied in clinical trials of curcumin. Various studies investigated the benefit of taking curcumin for colorectal cancer patients, one of the first of which was conducted by Cruz-Correa *et al*. Five familial adenomatous polyposis (FAP) patients (3 men and 2 women) with previous colectomy (4 with ileorectal anastomosis and 1 with ileoanal pull through with ileal anal pouch) were included in the study. The patients received a combination of 440 mg curcumin and 20 mg of quercetin thrice daily. The parameters assessed in this study were the number and size of polyps in each patient. The mean treatment duration was 6 months, with a range of 3-9 months. It was found that one patient was non-compliant in months 3 to 6 and one patient was lost to follow-up after 3 months of treatment. The first patient was reinstructed with the correct regiment and continued the therapy to month 9. Both patients were included in the analysis since the number of patients was limited in this study. All 5 patients had a significant decrease ($P < 0.05$) in the number (60.4%) and size (50.9%) of polyps compared to the baseline. Since both curcumin and quercetin were used in this study, it cannot be concluded that curcumin alone is beneficial in colorectal patients. More studies are needed to confirm the efficacy of curcumin [41].

The first study that evaluated the benefit of administration of lone curcumin to colorectal cancer patients was conducted by Sharma *et al*. A total of 15 patients with advanced colorectal cancer refractory to standard chemotherapies were included in this study. Curcumin mentioned in this study referred to 500 mg capsules containing 450 mg of curcumin, 40 mg of desmethoxycurcumin and 10 mg of bisdesmethoxycurcumin confirmed by HPLC/MS. All patients received curcumin 0.45 – 3.6 g (1 – 8 capsules) once daily for up to 4 months. Two patients showed stable disease by radiologic criteria after 2 months of treatment and this condition remained for 4 months. From the aspect of quality of life score, 1 patient noticed a significant improvement after 1 month of treatment while 2 patients' condition became worse, as confirmed by them having radiologic progressive disease. Consumption of curcumin 3.6 g daily resulted in 62% (day 1) and 57% (day 29) decrease in inducible PGE2 production in blood samples taken 1 hour after dose administration on the aforementioned days. Both results showed a significant decrease ($P < 0.05$) compared to the baseline [42].

Caroll *et al*. Conducted another study involving curcumin and colorectal cancer, a phase II clinical trial. The study was a non-randomized, open-label clinical trial in 44 eligible smokers with 8 or more rectal aberrant crypt foci (ACF) on screening colonoscopy. The micronized curcumin was given orally 2 g (8 capsules) once daily at the first stage and 4 g (16 capsules) once daily in the second stage, with each stage using different patients. Pre- and post-treatment concentrations of prostaglandin E2 (PGE2) and 5-hydroxyeicosatetraenoic acid (5-HETE) in ACF and normal-tissue biopsies were measured. This study showed that neither doses of curcumin reduced PGE2 or 5-HETE within ACF or normal mucosa. Curcumin 4 mg showed a significant 40% reduction in ACF number ($P < 0.005$), but the same result was not observed in the 2 g group [43].

Another study was performed by He *et al*., on 126 patients with colorectal cancer (63 patients received curcumin and 63 patients received a vehicle as the control group). This study was a randomized, double-blind study. The results showed that the administration of 360 mg curcumin capsule thrice/day during the period ahead of surgery with treatment duration varied between 10 to 30 days significantly improved patients' body weight after 10 days of treatment (P< 0.05) compared to the control group. Furthermore, the study concluded that the administration of curcumin decreases TNF-α and Bcl-2 levels, speeds up cancer cell apoptosis and increases the expression of p53 and levels of Bax in colorectal cancer [44].

Pancreatic Cancer

One of the first studies conducted to evaluate the benefit of curcumin on pancreatic cancer was performed by Dhillon *et al*. This study was a non-randomized, open-label, phase II trial of curcumin. A total of 25 patients who had histologically confirmed adenocarcinoma of the pancreas were included in this study. Patients were given 8 g curcumin daily until disease progression. Curcumin was given in the form of 1 g caplets containing 900 mg curcumin, 80 mg desmethoxycurcumin, and 20 mg bisdesmethoxycurcumin. Patient conditions, including the disease progression, were evaluated every 2 months. Serum cytokine levels for interleukin (IL)-6, IL-8, IL-10, and IL-1 receptor antagonists and peripheral blood mononuclear cell expression of NF-kappaB and cyclooxygenase-2 were monitored. Of the 25 patients, only 21 were evaluable for response; two patients showed clinical, biological activity, one patient remained stable with no disease progression for more than 18 months, and another patient had a dramatic but brief tumor response. The first patient who had a stable condition for more than 18 months showed slow improvement over 1.5 years and had decreases in all cytokine levels. The second patient showed a marked tumor regression (73%) accompanied by significant increases (4- to 35-fold) in serum cytokine levels (IL-6, IL-8, IL-10, and IL-1 receptor antagonists). The authors did not mention in detail the condition of the rest of the participants in this study and did not perform any statistical analysis to compare the patient conditions pre- and post-treatment of curcumin. Similar to most studies, there was considerable interindividual variation in plasma curcumin levels, and drug levels peaked at 22 to 41 ng/mL [45].

A second study involving pancreatic cancer was conducted by Epelbaum *et al.*, which evaluated the benefit of curcumin in combination with gemcitabine on pancreatic cancer patients. Seventeen patients (10 men and 7 women) with locally advanced tumor (n= 6) and metastatic disease (n= 11) were included in this study. All patients received curcumin 8 g once daily with gemcitabine 1000 mg/m^2 IV weekly × 3 out of 4 weeks. Five patients discontinued curcumin within 2 weeks of administration due to intractable abdominal fullness or pain. The rest of the patients took curcumin for 1 – 12 months. Curcumin dose was reduced to 4 g/day in some patients because of abdominal pain. The clinical response from 11 evaluable patients showed that 1 patient (9%) had a partial response for 7 months, 4 patients (36%) had stable disease (2, 3, 6, and 12 months progression-free survival) and 6 patients had tumor progression. TTP was 1 to 12 months with a median of 2 months and overall survival of 1 to 24 months with a median of 6 months. There was no comparison with the sole administration of gemcitabine in this study, so the benefit of curcumin for pancreatic cancer patients remains unconcluded [46].

A similar study was performed by Kanai *et al.*, who evaluated a combination of gemcitabine and curcumin for pancreatic cancer. The study was a phase 1/2 open-label study. A total of 21 patients with advanced pancreatic cancer who showed disease progression during gemcitabine-based chemotherapy were included in this study. Patients received a combination of intravenous gemcitabine at a dose of 1,000 mg/m^2 on days 1 and 8 and 60 mg/m^2 of S-1 orally for 14 consecutive days every 3 weeks and curcumin 8 g daily. Curcumin was given in the form of a microbead consisting of a mixture of curcuminoids (curcumin 73%, demethoxycurcumin 22%, and bisdemethoxycurcumin 4%). The median survival time after curcumin administration was 161 days (95% confidence interval 109-223 days) and the 1-year survival rate was 19% (4.4-41.4%). Similar to the previous study, there was no comparison with the lone administration of gemcitabine in this study [47].

Prostate Cancer

A study conducted by Ide *et al.* determined the effect of curcumin and isoflavones on prostate-specific antigen (PSA) levels in general, and not specific to prostate cancer. This study was a randomized placebo-controlled double-blind study. A total of 85 men were randomized to receive either a combination of curcumin 100 mg and isoflavones 40 mg (containing 66% daidzein, 24% glycitein, and 10% genistin), or placebo. PSA levels were evaluated before and 6 months after treatment. Both supplement and placebo groups did not show any differences in PSA levels between baseline and the end of treatment, but analysis of subgroups showed that the combination decreased PSA levels significantly in patients with PSA levels of more than 10. This study implied the prospect of curcumin in decreasing PSA levels in patients with prostate cancer [48].

Depression

Several studies have been conducted to evaluate the efficacy of curcumin towards patients with major depressive disorder. Lopresti *et al.*, conducted a randomized, double-blind, placebo-controlled study on patients with major depressive disorder. A total of 56 patients were randomized to receive curcumin 500 mg twice daily or placebo for 8 weeks. After 4 weeks, both groups showed improvement in the primary measure, the Inventory of Depressive Symptomatology self-rated version (IDS-SR$_{30}$), but after 8 weeks, curcumin was significantly more effective than the placebo in improving several mood-related symptoms. More promising results of curcumin treatment have been observed in a subgroup of patients with atypical depression [49].

In addition to monotherapy, Sanmukhani *et al.*, conducted a study on patients with major depressive disorder in a single-blind, randomized controlled trial involving fluoxetine, curcumin, and their combination. In this study, a total of 60 patients were randomized to receive fluoxetine 20 mg, and curcumin 1000 mg, or the combination of both for 6 weeks. The primary efficacy variable used in this study was response rates according to the Hamilton Depression Rating Scale, 17-item version (HAM-D17). After completion of the study, the percentage of responders was highest in the combination group (77.8%) but failed to show significant results statistically compared to fluoxetine (64.7%) and the curcumin (62.5%) groups. In this study, the benefit of curcumin was at least comparable to fluoxetine [50]. In another clinical study conducted by Bergman *et al.* administration of curcumin-escitalopram or curcumin-venlafaxine combinations for 5 weeks failed to show statistically significant improvements in the outcome measures compared to placebo [51]. Furthermore, a study by Yu *et al.* (n = 108) showed that the combination of curcumin 1000 mg and antidepressant for 6 weeks showed improvement in behavioral response, which was demonstrated by significantly reduced HAM-D17 and Montgomery-Asberg Depression Rating Scale scores. In addition, curcumin decreased the inflammatory cytokines interleukin 1β and tumor necrosis factor α levels, and plasma brain-derived neurotrophic factor levels, and decreased salivary cortisol concentrations compared with the placebo group [52].

Diabetes Mellitus

A study was performed by Usharani *et al.*, in patients with type 2 diabetes mellitus. The study was a randomized, parallel-group, placebo-controlled, 8-week study. A total of 72 patients with type 2 diabetes were randomized to receive NCB-02 (two capsules containing curcumin 150 mg twice daily), atorvastatin 10 mg once daily, or placebo for 8 weeks. Although the study was conducted on patients with type 2 diabetes, the main parameters evaluated in this study were endothelial function, oxidative stress, and inflammatory markers. There was a significant improvement in endothelial function after treatment with atorvastatin (-3.63 ± 3.17% *vs* -8.95 ± 6.80%) and NCB-02 (-2.69 ± 3.02% *vs* -8.19 ± 5.73%). Patients who received atorvastatin or NCB-02 also showed significant reductions in the levels of malondialdehyde, ET-1, IL-6, and TNF-α. Changes in the measured parameters of the placebo group were statistically insignificant [53].

Dyslipidemia

A study performed by Mohammadi *et al.* evaluated the effect of curcumin in lowering blood lipid levels in obese patients. The study was a randomized, double-blind, placebo-controlled, crossover trial. A total of 30 patients were randomized to receive curcuminoids 1 g/day or placebo for 30 days. The study concluded that curcuminoid administration resulted in a significant reduction of only serum triglycerides ($P = 0.009$), while total cholesterol, low-density lipoprotein cholesterol, high-density lipoprotein cholesterol, and high-sensitivity C-reactive protein remained unchanged. Anthropometric parameters, including weight, body-mass index, waist circumference, hip circumference, arm circumference, and body fat, also remained unchanged by the end of the study [54]. It was found that mean serum levels of IL-1β ($P = 0.042$), IL-4 ($P = 0.008$), and VEGF ($P = 0.01$) were significantly reduced by curcumin therapy. There were no significant changes observed in the concentrations of IL-2, IL-6, IL-8, IL-10, IFNγ, EGF, and MCP-1 [55].

In addition, Sahebkar *et al.* conducted a meta-analysis to assess the effect of curcumin on blood lipid levels. Only 5 studies met the selection criteria in this meta-analysis, including the previous study by Mohammadi *et al.* [54]. Other studies were not elaborated in detail in this review because of the inclusion criteria used in this study. While the study by Mohammadi *et al.* used obese dyslipidemia patients as the inclusion criteria, other studies used a different approach, such as elderly subjects with an established diagnosis of Alzheimer's disease [56], patients with acute coronary syndrome [57], patients with type 2 diabetes mellitus [53], and healthy subjects [58]. Hence, only the first study was reviewed in detail in this section, but other studies will be included as a part of the meta-analysis. The analysis showed that curcumin did not affect any lipid parameters compared to the control group. There was high variability in the effect of curcumin towards total cholesterol, LDL-C, and triglycerides, but not HDL-C. The result was expected to have a high variability because of the different inclusion criteria that affected the control groups used, which varied from placebo, vitamin E, to atorvastatin [59].

Inflammatory Bowel Disease

A small pilot study on curcumin therapy in inflammatory bowel disease was conducted by Holt *et al*. Ten subjects diagnosed with ulcerative proctitis or proctosigmoiditis (n= 5) or Crohn's disease (n= 5) were included in this study. The curcumin regiment was different for proctitis and Crohn's disease, but the authors did not state the reason.

Five patients with ulcerative proctitis or proctosigmoiditis (3 women and 2 men) were given 550 mg of curcumin twice daily for 1 month and then 550 mg three times daily for another month. All patients were evaluated for indexes of inflammation (sedimentation rate and C-reactive protein [CRP]) and had sigmoidoscopies and biopsies both at baseline and 2 months later when the study ended. All five subjects with proctitis showed significant improvement ($P < 0.02$) in global scores. However, despite this significant change in global scores, the findings were varied between the individuals; 2 subjects showed a 7 point decrease (improvement) in the global score and 3 patients showed 2-3 points decrease (improvement) in the global score.

For Crohn's disease, five patients (3 men and 2 women) were included in the study, but one subject did not complete this study. The subjects were given curcumin for 3 months. For the first month, curcumin 360 mg (1 capsule) was given three times daily and for the remaining two months, the regiment was changed to 360 mg (4 capsules) four times daily. All patients were evaluated for Crohn's Disease Activity Index (CDAI), CRP, erythrocyte sedimentation rate (ESR), complete blood counts, and liver and renal function. The CDAI decreased 12.9–38.7%, while the sedimentation rate decreased 17.4–70.8% in all patients. Similar to the results of the proctitis patients, these findings showed high variability between patients. A larger number of patients and a better study design is needed to confirm the efficacy of curcumin towards inflammatory bowel disease [60].

Moreover, in an *ex vivo* study conducted by Epstein *et al*., using colonic mucosal biopsies and colonic myofibroblasts (CMF) from children and adults with active IBD, curcumin showed the suppression of p38 mitogen-activated protein kinase activation, reduction of IL-1b and matrix metalloproteinase-3 and the increase of IL-10 [61].

Metabolic Syndrome (Weight Loss)

Not many studies that evaluated the effect of turmeric used weight reduction as the primary efficacy endpoint; usually, weight reduction was used as the secondary efficacy endpoint in addition to other parameters in metabolic syndrome. Hence, in this section, pooled data from a meta-analysis was used to review the effect of curcumin on weight loss.

Akbari *et al.*, performed a systematic review and meta-analysis of randomized controlled trials to assess the effect of curcumin in reducing weight among patients with metabolic syndrome and related disorders. As many as 18 articles (21 studies) were eligible to be evaluated in this study. Curcumin significantly reduced body mass index (BMI) ($P < 0.01$), weight ($P < 0.01$), waist-circumference (WC) ($P = 0.01$), leptin levels ($P < 0.001$) and increased adiponectin levels ($P = 0.01$), although no significant effect of curcumin intake on the hip ratio ($P = 0.18$) was observed in this analysis. There was significant heterogeneity among the included studies, which may be caused by different methodologies, dosage, formulation, duration, and population criteria of these studies [62].

Multiple Myeloma

A single-blind, cross-over pilot study performed by Golombick *et al.* on 26 patients (16 men and 10 women) with Monoclonal Gammopathy of Undefined Significance showed that the administration of oral curcumin 4 grams/day given as curcuminoid tablets decreased paraprotein load and urinary N-telopeptide of type I collagen. The clinical findings from Vadhan-Raj [63] confirmed that curcumin could downregulate NF-kB, STAT3, and COX2 in patients with multiple myeloma [64].

Pancreatitis

A pilot study of curcumin use for pancreatitis was conducted by Durgaprasad *et al.* on patients with tropical pancreatitis. A total of twenty-two patients were randomized into two groups, treatment for 6 weeks with a combination of 500 mg of curcumin with 5 mg of piperine, and placebo. The pattern of pain, and on red blood cell levels of malonyldialdehyde (MDA) and glutathione (GSH), were assessed in this study. There was a significant decrease in erythrocyte MDA levels and a significant increase in GSH levels on the curcumin-piperine group compared to the placebo [65]. Adding piperine into the curcumin regiment has been proven to increase curcumin bioavailability in humans [12].

Osteoarthritis

One of the clinical studies for osteoarthritis was conducted using a proprietary complex of curcumin with soy phosphatidylcholine (Meriva®, Indena SpA). A total of 50 patients with mild to moderate pain not adequately or completely controlled with anti-inflammatory drugs were included in this study. The subjects were divided into two groups: group A with the "best available treatment" and group B with the "best available treatment and Meriva". Curcumin was given as Meriva® 1000 mg capsules (natural curcuminoid mixture (20%), phosphatidylcholine (40%), and microcrystalline cellulose (40%)), equivalent to 200 mg curcuminoid, per day. The composition of the curcuminoid mixture was 75% curcumin, 15% demethoxycurcumin, and 10% bisdemethoxycurcumin. Osteoarthritis (OA) signs/symptoms were evaluated using Western Ontario and McMaster Universities (WOMAC) scores and mobility was evaluated by walking performance on a treadmill. After 3 months of curcumin administration, there was a significant improvement in all patients. The authors stated that the global WOMAC score decreased by 58% (P<0.05) and walking distance in the treadmill test was prolonged from 76 m to 332 m (P<0.05). In addition, the overall treatment cost (medication, treatment, and hospitalization) was reduced significantly in the treatment group [65]. Although this study showed positive results, the study design was confusing and potentially led to misleading results because what was considered as "best available treatment" remained unclear and the patient dispositions were not mentioned [66].

The previous study was continued by Belcaro *et al.*, for a longer period of time, since OA is a chronic condition that usually requires lifelong treatment. This study used the same product as the previous study, but was conducted over 8 months and involved 100 patients. The clinical endpoints were the WOMAC score, Karnofsky Performance Scale Index, and treadmill walking performance. This study used the same study design as the previous study. Curcumin, given as Meriva capsules, significantly improved the Karnofsky Scale from 73.3 to 92.2 ($P < 0.05$), decreased the scores for pain from 16.6 to 7.3 ($P < 0.05$), reduced the score of stiffness from 7.4 to 3.2 ($P < 0.05$), decreased the global WOMAC score from 80.6 to 33.3 ($P < 0.05$), and increased the distance of the treadmill test from 77.3 to 344 meters ($P < 0.05$). All the mentioned parameters showed insignificant changes for subjects in the control group [67].

Rheumatoid Arthritis

Curcumin is widely acknowledged to have anti-inflammatory properties. In relation to this, a pilot study was conducted by Chandran *et al.*, to evaluate the safety and efficacy of curcumin toward patients with rheumatoid arthritis (RA). A total of 45 patients (38 females, 7 male) with active RA (RA functional class I or II) and Disease Activity Score (DAS) > 5.1) were included for an 8-week study. The study was a randomized, single-blinded, pilot study. The patients were divided into 3 arms in this study: patients receiving curcumin capsule 500 mg, diclofenac sodium 50 mg, and their combination. Curcumin was given in the form of BCM-95W (a patented and registered formulation of curcumin with enhanced bioavailability). All treatment groups showed statistically significant changes in Disease Activity Score (DAS) scores, including the curcumin group, which showed the highest overall DAS scores, along with the American College of Rheumatology (ACR) criteria for an overall reduction in tenderness and swelling of joint scores. The curcumin group showed comparable results with the diclofenac sodium group in all parameters [68].

Skin Diseases

Curcumin has demonstrated a beneficial effect on skin diseases, such as pruritis, psoriasis, and vitiligo. The first study evaluated the effect of curcumin in alleviating sulfur mustard (SM) induced chronic pruritic symptoms. This study was a randomized, double-blind, placebo-controlled study. A total of 96 male Iranian veterans were randomized to receive curcumin 1 g/day (n = 46) or placebo (n = 50) for 4 weeks. The efficacy of curcumin was evaluated using the pruritus score, visual analog scale (VAS), and scoring atopic dermatitis (SCORAD) index. The quality of life was also evaluated using the Dermatology Life Quality Index (DLQI) questionnaire. Curcumin significantly reduced serum concentrations of substance P ($P < 0.001$), activities of superoxide dismutase ($P = 0.02$), glutathione peroxidase ($P = 0.006$), and catalase ($P < 0.001$). Curcumin also demonstrated significant reduction in pruritus severity, including the pruritus score ($P < 0.001$), VAS score ($P < 0.001$), overall ($P < 0.001$) and objective SCORAD ($P = 0.009$), and DLQI's first question ($P < 0.001$). None of these measures were significantly changed in the placebo group [69]. Further studies need to be conducted, especially towards different causes of pruritus, in order to draw a definite conclusion.

One of the first studies that evaluated the effect of curcumin on skin disease was conducted by Kurd *et al.* The study was a phase II, open-label, Simon's two-stage study. A total of 12 patients with plaque psoriasis were included to receive 4.5 g/day of oral curcuminoid C3 complex. Only 2 patients counted as responders with improvement in the Psoriasis Area and Severity Index (PSAI). However, the results were questionable due to the small sample size and the absence of a control group [70]. This limitation was improved in a randomized, placebo-control clinical trial conducted by Bahraini *et al*. A total of 40 patients with scalp psoriasis were randomized to receive turmeric tonic twice a day or placebo for 9 weeks. In this study, turmeric tonic significantly reduced the erythema, scaling, and induration of lesions (PASI score), and improved the patients' quality of life ($P < 0.05$) compared to placebo [71]. It was suggested that curcumin showed a positive effect in improving the condition in patients with psoriasis by reducing PhK (serin/threonine-specific protein kinase) activity and keratinocyte transferrin receptor (TRR) expression, reducing parakeratosis severity and epidermal CD8+ cells density, and reducing IL-22 [72, 73].

Lastly, a preliminary randomized controlled study was conducted by Asawanonda and Klahan in patients with focal or generalized vitiligo. A total of 10 patients were randomized to receive targeted narrowband UVB plus topical tetrahydrocurcuminoid cream, or targeted UVB alone, for 12 weeks. After completion of the study, both treatment groups showed significant repigmentation compared to baseline. The treatment group did not show significant improvement when compared to the placebo, implying that UVB alone is enough for the treatment of vitiligo [74].

Viral Infection

A simple clinical trial was conducted by James to evaluate curcumin as an antiviral agent in 40 patients with HIV. The parameters examined in this study were viral load tests following low and high dose regiments of curcumin. This study showed that curcumin did not affect viral load or CD4 counts in patients [75].

SUMMARY OF CLINICAL TRIAL

A summary of clinical trials of turmeric, turmeric-based medicine, and turmeric isolate is presented in Table **1**.

ADVERSE EFFECT IN CLINICAL TRIALS

In most clinical trials, both turmeric and curcumin proved to be safe and well-tolerated in most patients. In some countries, such as the United States,, curcumin is categorized as "Generally Recognized as Safe" (GRAS) by the Food and Drug Administration (FDA) [76]. National regulatory bodies in other countries, however, such as Belgium's Federal Agency for Food Chain Safety and Italy's National Institute of Health, have issued a warning to consumers for certain turmeric supplements that were associated with a sudden increase of acute cholestatic hepatitis [77].

Table 1. A summary of clinical trials of turmeric.

S.No	Disease/ Condition	Number of Subjects	Study Design	Regiment and Formulation	Results	Ref
**Turmeric and Turmeric-based Medicine**
1	Arthritis	107	Randomized, controlled, active comparator	Turmeric extract 2 g daily for 6 weeks	Turmeric significantly improved the patient's condition in pain on level walking, pain on stairs, and functions of the knee at weeks 2, 4, and 6. The result was comparable to ibuprofen 800 mg.	[14]
		120	Randomized, single-blind, placebo-controlled	Polysaccharide-rich turmeric extract 500 mg twice daily for 42 days	Post-treatments scores using VAS, WOMAC, and CGIC, assessed on day 21 and 42 showed significant improvement compared to placebo.	[15]
		150	Randomized, double-blind, multicenter, placebo-controlled	Bio-optimized *Curcuma longa* extract (BCL), low dose (2 x 46.67 turmeric extract) or high dose (3 x 46.67 turmeric extract) for 3 months	No significant results for PGAD and sColl-2-1. Significantly decreased knee pain on the VAS score.	[16]
2	Asthma	55	Randomized, double-blind, placebo-controlled	Turmeric powder 30 mg/kg/day of for 6 months or placebo on top of the standard therapy	No significant results for all parameters.	[18]
3	Chemoprevention	22	Not mentioned	Turmeric tablet 1.5 g daily for 30 days	Turmeric significantly reduced the urinary excretion of mutagens in smokers.	[19]

(Table 1) cont.....

S.No	Disease/ Condition	Number of Subjects	Study Design	Regiment and Formulation	Results	Ref
				Turmeric and Turmeric-based Medicine		
4	Colorectal cancer	15	Pilot study	Turmeric extract 440 – 2200 mg daily for up to 4 months	Patients who were taking 440 mg turmeric extract for 29 days showed a 59% decrease in lymphocytic glutathione S-transferase activity. The effect was not observed at a higher dose.	[20]
5	Diabetes Mellitus	35	Randomized, double-blind, parallel study	Combination of turmeric 1200 mg and allium extract 1200 mg daily for 14 weeks	The combination significantly decreased fasting blood glucose, 2 hours postprandial blood glucose, and HbA1C. The result was comparable with glibenclamide 5 mg.	[21]
6	Dyslipidemia	32	Randomized, double-blind, parallel study	Combination of turmeric and garlic 1200, 1600, and 2400 mg daily for 14 weeks	No significant decrease in total cholesterol, LDL, and triglycerides on dyslipidemia patients with diabetes mellitus	[23]
		39	Randomized, double-blind, parallel study	Combination of 1200 mg turmeric and 1200 mg allium extract daily for 12 weeks	The results showed comparable results with simvastatin 5 mg in overall lipid profile analysis.	[24]
7	Human Gut Microbiota	14	Randomized, double-blind, placebo-controlled pilot study	Turmeric-piperine or curcumine-piperine once	Turmeric group showed a 7% increase and curcumin showed a 69% increase in detected species compared to the placebo group that showed a 15% reduction in detected species post-treatment.	[26]
8	Lupus nephritis	24	Randomized and placebo-controlled study	Turmeric 500 mg daily for 3 months	No significant result for all parameters.	[27]

(Table 1) cont.....

S.No	Disease/ Condition	Number of Subjects	Study Design	Regiment and Formulation	Results	Ref
				Turmeric and Turmeric-based Medicine		
9	Peptic ulcer	130	Randomized, double-blind, placebo-controlled study	Turmeric tablets 6 g daily for 8 weeks	No significant result for all parameters.	[28]
		45	Open-labeled, pilot study	Turmeric 3 g daily for 8 weeks	Ulcers were absent in 48% (12 DU and GU 3) patients after 4 weeks of treatment. This number increased to 72% (DU 13 and GU 5) after 8 weeks of treatment and 76% after 12 weeks (DU 14 and GU 5).	[29]
9	Skin Inflammation	47	Randomized, double-blind, placebo-controlled	Daily hot water extract of turmeric with or without curcumin for 4-8 weeks	The turmeric administration significantly increased the water content of the face after 4-8 weeks of treatment compared to the placebo, but failed to show a significant difference in trans-epidermal water loss and minimal erythema	[30]
10	Vascular function	136	Randomized, double-blind, placebo-controlled	Turmeric 400 mg thrice daily for 90 days	Turmeric showed a significant reduction from baseline in carotid–femoral pulse wave velocity, left brachial–ankle pulse wave velocity, aortic augmentation pressure, aortic augmentation index, and aortic augmentation index at heart rate 75 compared to the placebo group	[31]

(Table 1) cont.....

S.No	Disease/ Condition	Number of Subjects	Study Design	Regiment and Formulation	Results	Ref
			Turmeric Isolates (Curcumin)			
1	Alzheimer's Disease	34	Randomized, placebo-controlled, double-blind, pilot study	Curcumin 1 g or 4 g, once daily combined with 1 capsule (120 mg) of standardized ginkgo leaf extract or placebo for 6 months	No difference in MMSE scores between curcumin and placebo, but there was an increase in plasma Aβ40 levels	[35]
		36	Randomized, placebo-controlled, double-blind continue to open label	Curcumin 2 g or 4 g once daily for 12 months	No difference was observed in MMSE ADAS-Cog NPI, and ADCS-ADL score, and biomarker levels between turmeric and placebo group	[36]
		96	Randomized, placebo-controlled, double-blind study	Biocurcumax™ (standardized extract of C. longa (88% curcuminoids and 7% volatile oil)) 1500 mg/day	No difference in clinical parameter compared to placebo	[37]
2	Beta-Thalassemia	21	Open-labeled, pilot study	Curcuminoid capsules 500 mg of daily for 12 months	Curcumin decreased significantly MDA, RBC SOD, RBC GSH-Px, RBC GSH, and NTBI serum after 6 months of treatment	[39]
3	Breast cancer	14	Open-labeled, pilot study	Curcumin capsules 500 – 8000 mg/day and docetaxel infusion 100 mg/m2 for six cycles of therapy	No progressive disease was observed on evaluable patients. The biological response showed up to 50% decrease in tumor marker in 4 patients. The maximum tolerated dose for curcumin was 6000 mg/day	[40]

(Table 1) cont.....

S.No	Disease/ Condition	Number of Subjects	Study Design	Regiment and Formulation	Results	Ref
				Turmeric Isolates (Curcumin)		
4	Colorectal cancer	5	Open-labeled, pilot study	Curcumin capsules 40 mg and quercetin 20 mg thrice daily for up to 9 months	All patients had a significant decrease in polyp number and size compared to the baseline	[41]
		15	Open-labeled, pilot study	Curcuminoid capsules 450 – 3600 mg daily for up to 4 months	Two patients showed stable disease by radiologic criteria after 2 months of treatment. Curcumin decreased PGE2.	[42]
		45	Open-labeled study	Micronized curcumin in capsules was given orally 2 g daily at the first stage and 4 g daily at the second stage	Curcumin 4 mg showed a significant 40% reduction in ACF number, but not in PGE2 and 5-HETE.	[43]
		126	Randomized, double-blind, and placebo-controlled study	Curcumin capsules 1080 mg daily for 10 – 30 days	Curcumin significantly improved patients' body weight, decreased TNF-α and Bcl-2 levels, speed up cancer cell apoptosis, and increased the expression of p53 and levels of Bax in colorectal cancer	[44]

(Table 1) cont.....

S.No	Disease/ Condition	Number of Subjects	Study Design	Regiment and Formulation	Results	Ref
			Turmeric Isolates (Curcumin)			
5	Pancreatic Cancer	25	Open-labeled study	Curcumin caplets 8 g daily until disease progression	One patient remained stable with no disease progression for >18 months	[45]
		11	Open-labeled study	Curcumin capsules 8 g daily with gemcitabine 1000 mg/m2 IV weekly × 3 out of 4 weeks.	1 patient (9%) had a partial response for 7 months, 4 patients (36%) had stable disease (2, 3, 6, and 12 months progression-free survival) and 6 patients had tumor progression.	[46]
		21	Open-labeled study	Intravenous gemcitabine at the dose of 1,000 mg/m2 on days 1 and 8 and 60 mg/m2 of S-1 orally for 14 consecutive days every 3 weeks and curcumin 8 g daily. Curcumin was given in the form of microbead consisting mixture of curcuminoid	Median survival time after curcumin administration was 161 days (95% confidence interval 109-223 days) and 1-year survival rate was 19% (4.4-41.4%).	[47]
6	Prostate Cancer	85	Randomized, double-blind, and placebo-controlled study	Combination of curcumin 100 mg and isoflavones 40 mg (containing 66% daidzen, 24% glycitin, and 10% genistin)	The combination decreased PSA levels significantly in patients with PSA levels ≥ 10	[48]

(Table 1) cont.....

S.No	Disease/ Condition	Number of Subjects	Study Design	Regiment and Formulation	Results	Ref
				Turmeric Isolates (Curcumin)		
7	Depression	56	Randomized, double-blind, placebo-controlled study	Curcumin 500 mg twice daily for 8 weeks	After 8 weeks, curcumin was significantly more effective than a placebo in improving several mood-related symptoms. A better result of curcumin treatment has been observed in subgroup patients with atypical depression	[49]
		60	Randomized, single-blind, placebo-controlled study	Curcumin 1000 mg or combination of curcumin 1000 mg and fluoxetine 20 mg for 6 weeks	The percentage of responders was the highest in the combination group (77.8%) but failed to show significant results statistically compared to fluoxetine (64.7%) and the curcumin (62.5%) groups. In this study, the benefit of curcumin at least was comparable to fluoxetine.	[50]
		108	Randomized, double-blind, placebo-controlled study	Combination of curcumin 1000 mg and antidepressant for 6 weeks	Curcumin caused improvement in behavioral response. In addition, curcumin decreased inflammatory cytokines interleukin 1β, tumor necrosis factor α level, and plasma brain-derived neurotrophic factor levels and decreased salivary cortisol concentrations compared with the placebo group	[52]

(Table 1) cont.....

S.No	Disease/ Condition	Number of Subjects	Study Design	Regiment and Formulation	Results	Ref
			Turmeric Isolates (Curcumin)			
8	Diabetes Mellitus	72	Randomized, parallel-group, placebo-controlled	Two capsules containing curcumin 150 mg twice daily for 8 weeks	Significant reductions in the levels of malondialdehyde, ET-1, IL-6, and TNF-α. Glucose level was not evaluated	[53]
9	Dyslipidemia	30	Randomized, double-blind, placebo-controlled, crossover study	Curcuminoid 1 g/day for 30 days	Only serum triglycerides were significantly reduced, but total cholesterol, low-density lipoprotein cholesterol, high-density lipoprotein cholesterol, and high-sensitivity C-reactive protein remained unchanged. Anthropometric parameters remained unchanged during the study	[54]
10	Inflammatory Bowel Disease	10	Open-labeled, pilot study	Patients with ulcerative proctitis or proctosigmoiditis was given 550 mg of curcumin twice daily for 1 month and then 550 mg three times daily for another month. For patients with Crohn's disease, curcumin 360 mg (1 capsule) was given three times daily for the first month and for the rest two months 360 mg (4 capsules) four times daily.	All five subjects with proctitis showed significant improvement in global scores. The CDAI decreased 12.9 – 38.7%, while the sedimentation rate decreased 17.4 – 70.8% in all patients with Crohn's disease.	[60]
11	Multiple Myeloma	26	Single-blind, cross-over pilot study	Oral curcumin 4 grams/day	Curcumin can downregulate NF-kB, STAT3, and COX2 in patients with multiple myeloma	[64]

(Table 1) cont.....

S.No	Disease/ Condition	Number of Subjects	Study Design	Regiment and Formulation	Results	Ref
			Turmeric Isolates (Curcumin)			
12	Pancreatitis	22	Randomized, double-blind, and placebo-controlled study	Curcumin 500 mg with 5 mg of piperine daily for 6 weeks	There was a significant decrease in erythrocyte MDA levels and a significant increase in GSH levels on the curcumin-piperine group	[65]
13	Osteoarthritis	50	Open-label study, top-up with other treatment	Complex of curcumin with soy phosphatidylcholine (1000 mg) for 3 months	There was significant improvement from all patients. The overall treatment cost reduced significantly	[66]
		100	Open-label study, top-up with other treatment	Complex of curcumin with soy phosphatidylcholine (1000 mg) for 8 months	There was a significant improvement from all patients. The overall treatment cost reduced significantly	[67]
14	Rheumatoid arthritis	45	Randomized, single-blinded, pilot study	Curcumin capsule 500 mg, diclofenac sodium 50 mg, and the combination of both for 8 weeks. Curcumin was given in the form of BCM-95W (a patented and registered formulation of curcumin with enhanced bioavailability).	Curcumin group showed comparable results with the diclofenac sodium group in all parameters	[68]

(Table 1) cont.....

S.No	Disease/ Condition	Number of Subjects	Study Design	Regiment and Formulation	Results	Ref
			Turmeric Isolates (Curcumin)			
15	Skin Disease	96	Randomized, double-blind, placebo-controlled study	Curcumin 1 g/day for 4 weeks	Curcumin demonstrated significant reduction in pruritus severity.	[69]
		12	Open-labeled, pilot study	4.5 g/day of oral curcuminoid C3 complex	Only 2 patients counted as responders with improvement in Psoriasis Area and Severity Index (PSAI). There was no placebo group.	[70]
		40	Randomized, double-blind, placebo-control study	Turmeric tonic twice daily for 9 weeks	Turmeric tonic significantly reduced the erythema, scaling, and induration of lesions (PASI score), and improved the patients' quality of life compared to placebo in patient with scalp psoriasis	[71]
		10	Randomized, placebo-control, pilot study	Tetrahydrocurcuminoid cream combined with targeted UVB	Not significant compared to targeted UVB alone	[74]
16	Viral Infection	40	Open-labeled, pilot study	Low and high dose regiments of curcumin	Curcumin did not affect viral load or CD4 counts in HIV patients	[51]

Curcumin itself is known for tolerability and safety at high doses in humans. Very few subjects withdrew from clinical trials because of the side effects of turmeric or curcumin. In a study with gemcitabine-resistant patients with pancreatic cancer, patients could tolerate 8 g oral curcumin daily in combination with gemcitabine-based chemotherapy [10, 15]. Other clinical studies mentioned in the previous section also showed that turmeric and curcumin can be used for long term therapy with minimum side effects, with 12 months being the longest duration of a conducted clinical trial. In one of the earliest clinical studies of curcumin, curcumin was shown to be safe even at 12 g daily dose for 3 months [78]. Various studies based on clinical trials have shown that curcumin does not cause any adverse complications on liver and kidney function [79]. However, the effect of turmeric or curcumin in pregnancy or lactating women is unclear, but there is no report that the use of turmeric as a spice in pregnancy or lactating women causes any harm.

The adverse effects of turmeric and curcumin were found to be mainly dose-dependent. For curcumin, adverse effects were observed at a dose of 4 g or higher, due to which compliance is also reduced. The most frequent adverse effect was a gastrointestinal disturbance, which was usually mild and did not need medical treatment. Some notable adverse effects aside from gastrointestinal disturbance were inhibition of sperm motility *in vitro*, inhibition of Hepcidin synthesis, iron chelation, transient rises in liver enzymes, suppression of platelet aggregation, contact dermatitis, and urticaria, but these findings were inconsistent and were not always detected in clinical studies. In general, turmeric and curcumin can be considered as a safe and well-tolerated drug, but further studies need to be conducted to prove this claim.

CONSENT FOR PUBLICATION

Not applicable.

CONFLICT OF INTEREST

The authors confirm that there is no conflict of interest.

ACKNOWLEDGEMENTS

Declared none.

REFERENCES

[1]   World Health Organization. WHO guidelines for assessing quality of herbal medicines with reference to contaminants and residues.

[2]   WHO. World Health Organization. WHO traditional medicine strategy 2014–2023

[3]   Parveen A, Parveen B, Parveen R, Ahmad S. Challenges and guidelines for clinical trial of herbal drugs. Journal of pharmacy & bioallied sciences 2015; 7(4): 329-33.

[4]   Wallace TC. Twenty years of the dietary supplement health and education act-how should dietary supplements be regulated? J Nutr 2015; 145(8): 1683-6.
       [http://dx.doi.org/10.3945/jn.115.211102] [PMID: 26063064]

[5]   Badan Pengawas, Obat dan Makanan, Peraturan Kepala. Pengawas Obat dan Makanan Republik Indonesia Nomor 9 Tahun 2014 tentang Tata Laksana Persetujuan Uji Klinik 2014.

[6]   World Health Organization. WHO traditional medicine strategy: 2014-2023. World Health Organization 2013.

[7]   Vaughn AR, Branum A, Sivamani RK. Effects of turmeric (*Curcuma longa*) on skin health: A systematic review of the clinical evidence. Phytother Res 2016; 30(8): 1243-64.
       [http://dx.doi.org/10.1002/ptr.5640] [PMID: 27213821]

[8]   Govindarajan VS, Stahl WH. Turmeric--chemistry, technology, and quality. Crit Rev Food Sci Nutr 1980; 12(3): 199-301.
[http://dx.doi.org/10.1080/10408398009527278] [PMID: 6993103]

[9]   Li S, Yuan W, Deng G, Wang P, Yang P, Aggarwal BB. Chemical composition and product quality control of turmeric (*Curcuma longa* L.) Pharmaceutical Crops 2011; 2(1)

[10]   Gupta SC, Patchva S, Aggarwal BB. Therapeutic roles of curcumin: lessons learned from clinical trials. AAPS J 2013; 15(1): 195-218.
[http://dx.doi.org/10.1208/s12248-012-9432-8] [PMID: 23143785]

[11]   Ammon HP, Wahl MA. Pharmacology of *Curcuma longa*. Planta Med 1991; 57(1): 1-7.
[http://dx.doi.org/10.1055/s-2006-960004] [PMID: 2062949]

[12]   Prasad S, Tyagi AK, Aggarwal BB. Recent developments in delivery, bioavailability, absorption and metabolism of curcumin: the golden pigment from golden spice. Cancer Res Treat 2014; 46(1): 2-18.
[http://dx.doi.org/10.4143/crt.2014.46.1.2]

[13]   Hewlings SJ, Kalman DS. Curcumin: a review of its' effects on human health. Foods 2017; 6(10): 92.
[http://dx.doi.org/10.3390/foods6100092] [PMID: 29065496]

[14]   Madhu K, Chanda K, Saji MJ. Safety and efficacy of *Curcuma longa* extract in the treatment of painful knee osteoarthritis: a randomized placebo-controlled trial. Inflammopharmacology 2013; 21(2): 129-36.
[http://dx.doi.org/10.1007/s10787-012-0163-3] [PMID: 23242572]

[15]   Gupta SC, Patchva S, Koh W, Aggarwal BB. Discovery of curcumin, a component of golden spice, and its miraculous biological activities. Clin Exp Pharmacol Physiol 2012; 39(3): 283-99.
[http://dx.doi.org/10.1111/j.1440-1681.2011.05648.x] [PMID: 22118895]

[16]   Henrotin Y, Malaise M, Wittoek R, *et al.* Bio-optimized *Curcuma longa* extract is efficient on knee osteoarthritis pain: a double-blind multicenter randomized placebo controlled three-arm study. Arthritis Res Ther 2019; 21(1): 179.
[http://dx.doi.org/10.1186/s13075-019-1960-5] [PMID: 31351488]

[17]   Daily JW, Yang M, Park S. Efficacy of turmeric extracts and curcumin for alleviating the symptoms of joint arthritis: a systematic review and meta-analysis of randomized clinical trials. J Med Food 2016; 19(8): 717-29.
[http://dx.doi.org/10.1089/jmf.2016.3705] [PMID: 27533649]

[18]   Manarin G, Anderson D, Silva JME, *et al. Curcuma longa* L. ameliorates asthma control in children and adolescents: A randomized, double-blind, controlled trial. J Ethnopharmacol 2019; 238111882
[http://dx.doi.org/10.1016/j.jep.2019.111882] [PMID: 30991137]

[19]   Polasa K, Raghuram TC, Krishna TP, Krishnaswamy K. Effect of turmeric on urinary mutagens in smokers. Mutagenesis 1992; 7(2): 107-9.
[http://dx.doi.org/10.1093/mutage/7.2.107] [PMID: 1579064]

[20]   Sharma RA, McLelland HR, Hill KA, *et al.* Pharmacodynamic and pharmacokinetic study of oral Curcuma extract in patients with colorectal cancer. Clin Cancer Res 2001; 7(7): 1894-900.
[PMID: 11448902]

[21]   Sukandar EY, Sudjana P, Adnyana IK, Setiawan AS, Yuniarni U. Recent study of turmeric in combination with garlic as antidiabetic agent. Procedia Chem 2014; 13: 44-56.
[http://dx.doi.org/10.1016/j.proche.2014.12.005]

[22]   Wickenberg J, Ingemansson SL, Hlebowicz J. Effects of *Curcuma longa* (turmeric) on postprandial plasma glucose and insulin in healthy subjects. Nutr J 2010; 9(1): 43.
[http://dx.doi.org/10.1186/1475-2891-9-43] [PMID: 20937162]

[23]   Sukandar EY, Permana H, Adnyana IK, *et al.* Clinical study of turmeric (*Curcuma longa* L.) and garlic (Allium sativum L.) extracts as antihyperglycemic and antihyperlipidemic agent in type-2

diabetes-dyslipidemia patients. Int J Pharmacol 2010; 6(4): 456-63.
[http://dx.doi.org/10.3923/ijp.2010.456.463]

[24]   Sukandar EY, Sigit JI, Leliqia NPE, Lestari F. Safety of Garlic (Allium Sativum) and Turmeric. J Med Sci 2013; 13(1): 10-8.
[http://dx.doi.org/10.3923/jms.2013.10.18]

[25]   Qin S, Huang L, Gong J, *et al.* Efficacy and safety of turmeric and curcumin in lowering blood lipid levels in patients with cardiovascular risk factors: a meta-analysis of randomized controlled trials. Nutr J 2017; 16(1): 68.
[http://dx.doi.org/10.1186/s12937-017-0293-y] [PMID: 29020971]

[26]   Peterson CT, Vaughn AR, Sharma V, *et al.* Effects of turmeric and curcumin dietary supplementation on human gut microbiota: A double-blind, randomized, placebo-controlled pilot study. J Evid Based Integr Med 2018; 23(Jan-Dec)X18790725
[http://dx.doi.org/10.1177/2515690X18790725] [PMID: 30088420]

[27]   Khajehdehi P, Zanjaninejad B, Aflaki E, *et al.* Oral supplementation of turmeric decreases proteinuria, hematuria, and systolic blood pressure in patients suffering from relapsing or refractory lupus nephritis: a randomized and placebo-controlled study. J Ren Nutr 2012; 22(1): 50-7.
[http://dx.doi.org/10.1053/j.jrn.2011.03.002] [PMID: 21742514]

[28]   Van Dau N, Ham NN, Khac DH, *et al.* The effects of a traditional drug, turmeric (*Curcuma longa*), and placebo on the healing of duodenal ulcer. Phytomedicine 1998; 5(1): 29-34.
[http://dx.doi.org/10.1016/S0944-7113(98)80056-1] [PMID: 23195696]

[29]   Prucksunand C, Indrasukhsri B, Leethochawalit M, Hungspreugs K. Phase II clinical trial on effect of the long turmeric (*Curcuma longa* Linn) on healing of peptic ulcer. Southeast Asian J Trop Med Public Health 2001; 32(1): 208-15.
[PMID: 11485087]

[30]   Asada K, Ohara T, Muroyama K, Yamamoto Y, Murosaki S. Effects of hot water extract of *Curcuma longa* on human epidermal keratinocytes *in vitro* and skin conditions in healthy participants: A randomized, double-blind, placebo-controlled trial. J Cosmet Dermatol 2019; 18(6): 1866-74.
[http://dx.doi.org/10.1111/jocd.12890] [PMID: 30809971]

[31]   Srinivasan A, Selvarajan S, Kamalanathan S, Kadhiravan T, Prasanna Lakshmi NC, Adithan S. Effect of *Curcuma longa* on vascular function in native Tamilians with type 2 diabetes mellitus: A randomized, double-blind, parallel arm, placebo-controlled trial. Phytother Res 2019; 33(7): 1898-911.
[http://dx.doi.org/10.1002/ptr.6381] [PMID: 31155769]

[32]   Maheshwari RK, Singh AK, Gaddipati J, Srimal RC. Multiple biological activities of curcumin: a short review. Life Sci 2006; 78(18): 2081-7.
[http://dx.doi.org/10.1016/j.lfs.2005.12.007] [PMID: 16413584]

[33]   Nagpal M, Sood S. Role of curcumin in systemic and oral health: An overview. J Nat Sci Biol Med 2013; 4(1): 3-7.
[http://dx.doi.org/10.4103/0976-9668.107253] [PMID: 23633828]

[34]   Sharma RA, Steward WP, Gescher AJ. Pharmacokinetics and pharmacodynamics of curcumin The molecular targets and therapeutic uses of curcumin in health and disease. Boston, MA: Springer 2007; pp. 453-70.
[http://dx.doi.org/10.1007/978-0-387-46401-5_20]

[35]   Baum L, Lam CW, Cheung SK, *et al.* Six-month randomized, placebo-controlled, double-blind, pilot clinical trial of curcumin in patients with Alzheimer disease. J Clin Psychopharmacol 2008; 28(1): 110-3.
[http://dx.doi.org/10.1097/jcp.0b013e318160862c] [PMID: 18204357]

[36]   Ringman JM, Frautschy SA, Teng E, *et al.* Oral curcumin for Alzheimer's disease: tolerability and efficacy in a 24-week randomized, double blind, placebo-controlled study. Alzheimers Res Ther 2012; 4(5): 43.

[http://dx.doi.org/10.1186/alzrt146] [PMID: 23107780]

[37]   Rainey-Smith SR, Brown BM, Sohrabi HR, *et al.* Curcumin and cognition: a randomised, placebo-controlled, double-blind study of community-dwelling older adults. Br J Nutr 2016; 115(12): 2106-13.
[http://dx.doi.org/10.1017/S0007114516001203] [PMID: 27102361]

[38]   Small GW, Siddarth P, Li Z, *et al.* Memory and brain amyloid and tau effects of a bioavailable form of curcumin in non-demented adults: a double-blind, placebo-controlled 18-month trial. Am J Geriatr Psychiatry 2018; 26(3): 266-77.
[http://dx.doi.org/10.1016/j.jagp.2017.10.010] [PMID: 29246725]

[39]   Kalpravidh RW, Siritanaratkul N, Insain P, *et al.* Improvement in oxidative stress and antioxidant parameters in β-thalassemia/Hb E patients treated with curcuminoids. Clin Biochem 2010; 43(4-5): 424-9.
[http://dx.doi.org/10.1016/j.clinbiochem.2009.10.057] [PMID: 19900435]

[40]   Bayet-Robert M, Kwiatkowski F, Leheurteur M, *et al.* Phase I dose escalation trial of docetaxel plus curcumin in patients with advanced and metastatic breast cancer. Cancer Biol Ther 2010; 9(1): 8-14.
[http://dx.doi.org/10.4161/cbt.9.1.10392] [PMID: 19901561]

[41]   Cruz-Correa M, Shoskes DA, Sanchez P, *et al.* Combination treatment with curcumin and quercetin of adenomas in familial adenomatous polyposis. Clin Gastroenterol Hepatol 2006; 4(8): 1035-8.
[http://dx.doi.org/10.1016/j.cgh.2006.03.020] [PMID: 16757216]

[42]   Sharma RA, Euden SA, Platton SL, *et al.* Phase I clinical trial of oral curcumin: biomarkers of systemic activity and compliance. Clin Cancer Res 2004; 10(20): 6847-54.
[http://dx.doi.org/10.1158/1078-0432.CCR-04-0744] [PMID: 15501961]

[43]   Carroll RE, Benya RV, Turgeon DK, *et al.* Phase IIa clinical trial of curcumin for the prevention of colorectal neoplasia. Cancer Prev Res (Phila) 2011; 4(3): 354-64.
[http://dx.doi.org/10.1158/1940-6207.CAPR-10-0098] [PMID: 21372035]

[44]   He ZY, Shi CB, Wen H, Li FL, Wang BL, Wang J. Upregulation of p53 expression in patients with colorectal cancer by administration of curcumin. Cancer Invest 2011; 29(3): 208-13.
[http://dx.doi.org/10.3109/07357907.2010.550592] [PMID: 21314329]

[45]   Dhillon N, Aggarwal BB, Newman RA, *et al.* Phase II trial of curcumin in patients with advanced pancreatic cancer. Clin Cancer Res 2008; 14(14): 4491-9.
[http://dx.doi.org/10.1158/1078-0432.CCR-08-0024] [PMID: 18628464]

[46]   Epelbaum R, Vizel B, Bar-Sela G. Phase II study of curcumin and gemcitabine in patients with advanced pancreatic cancer. Journal of Clinical Oncology 2008; 26(15_suppl): 15619.
[http://dx.doi.org/10.1200/jco.2008.26.15_suppl.15619]

[47]   Kanai M, Yoshimura K, Asada M, *et al.* A phase I/II study of gemcitabine-based chemotherapy plus curcumin for patients with gemcitabine-resistant pancreatic cancer. Cancer Chemother Pharmacol 2011; 68(1): 157-64.
[http://dx.doi.org/10.1007/s00280-010-1470-2] [PMID: 20859741]

[48]   Ide H, Tokiwa S, Sakamaki K, *et al.* Combined inhibitory effects of soy isoflavones and curcumin on the production of prostate-specific antigen. Prostate 2010; 70(10): 1127-33.
[http://dx.doi.org/10.1002/pros.21147] [PMID: 20503397]

[49]   Lopresti AL, Maes M, Maker GL, Hood SD, Drummond PD. Curcumin for the treatment of major depression: a randomised, double-blind, placebo controlled study. J Affect Disord 2014; 167: 368-75.
[http://dx.doi.org/10.1016/j.jad.2014.06.001] [PMID: 25046624]

[50]   Sanmukhani J, Satodia V, Trivedi J, *et al.* Efficacy and safety of curcumin in major depressive disorder: a randomized controlled trial. Phytother Res 2014; 28(4): 579-85.
[http://dx.doi.org/10.1002/ptr.5025] [PMID: 23832433]

[51]   Bergman J, Miodownik C, Bersudsky Y, *et al.* Curcumin as an add-on to antidepressive treatment: a randomized, double-blind, placebo-controlled, pilot clinical study. Clin Neuropharmacol 2013; 36(3):

73-7.
[http://dx.doi.org/10.1097/WNF.0b013e31828ef969] [PMID: 23673908]

[52]   Yu JJ, Pei LB, Zhang Y, Wen ZY, Yang JL. Chronic supplementation of curcumin enhances the efficacy of antidepressants in major depressive disorder: a randomized, double-blind, placebo-controlled pilot study. J Clin Psychopharmacol 2015; 35(4): 406-10.
[http://dx.doi.org/10.1097/JCP.0000000000000352] [PMID: 26066335]

[53]   Usharani P, Mateen AA, Naidu MU, Raju YS, Chandra N. Effect of NCB-02, atorvastatin and placebo on endothelial function, oxidative stress and inflammatory markers in patients with type 2 diabetes mellitus: a randomized, parallel-group, placebo-controlled, 8-week study. Drugs R D 2008; 9(4): 243-50.
[http://dx.doi.org/10.2165/00126839-200809040-00004] [PMID: 18588355]

[54]   Mohammadi A, Sahebkar A, Iranshahi M, *et al.* Effects of supplementation with curcuminoids on dyslipidemia in obese patients: a randomized crossover trial. Phytother Res 2013; 27(3): 374-9.
[http://dx.doi.org/10.1002/ptr.4715] [PMID: 22610853]

[55]   Ganjali S, Sahebkar A, Mahdipour E, *et al.* Investigation of the effects of curcumin on serum cytokines in obese individuals: a randomized controlled trial. The Scientific World Journal 2014; 2014
[http://dx.doi.org/10.1155/2014/898361]

[56]   Baum L, Cheung SK, Mok VC, *et al.* Curcumin effects on blood lipid profile in a 6-month human study. Pharmacol Res 2007; 56(6): 509-14.
[http://dx.doi.org/10.1016/j.phrs.2007.09.013] [PMID: 17951067]

[57]   Alwi I, Santoso T, Suyono S, *et al.* The effect of curcumin on lipid level in patients with acute coronary syndrome. Acta Med Indones 2008; 40(4): 201-10.
[PMID: 19151449]

[58]   Pungcharoenkul K, Thongnopnua P. Effect of different curcuminoid supplement dosages on total *in vivo* antioxidant capacity and cholesterol levels of healthy human subjects. Phytother Res 2011; 25(11): 1721-6.
[http://dx.doi.org/10.1002/ptr.3608] [PMID: 21796707]

[59]   Sahebkar A. A systematic review and meta-analysis of randomized controlled trials investigating the effects of curcumin on blood lipid levels. Clin Nutr 2014; 33(3): 406-14.
[http://dx.doi.org/10.1016/j.clnu.2013.09.012] [PMID: 24139527]

[60]   Holt PR, Katz S, Kirshoff R. Curcumin therapy in inflammatory bowel disease: a pilot study. Dig Dis Sci 2005; 50(11): 2191-3.
[http://dx.doi.org/10.1007/s10620-005-3032-8] [PMID: 16240238]

[61]   Epstein J, Docena G, MacDonald TT, Sanderson IR. Curcumin suppresses p38 mitogen-activated protein kinase activation, reduces IL-1β and matrix metalloproteinase-3 and enhances IL-10 in the mucosa of children and adults with inflammatory bowel disease. Br J Nutr 2010; 103(6): 824-32.
[http://dx.doi.org/10.1017/S0007114509992510] [PMID: 19878610]

[62]   Akbari M, Lankarani KB, Tabrizi R, *et al.* The effects of curcumin on weight loss among patients with metabolic syndrome and related disorders: a systematic review and meta-analysis of randomized controlled trials. Front Pharmacol 2019; 10: 649.
[http://dx.doi.org/10.3389/fphar.2019.00649] [PMID: 31249528]

[63]   Vadhan-Raj S, Weber DM, Wang M, *et al.* Curcumin downregulates NF-kB and related genes in patients with multiple myeloma: results of a phase I/II study. Blood 2007; 110(11): 1177.
[http://dx.doi.org/10.1182/blood.V110.11.1177.1177]

[64]   Golombick T, Diamond TH, Badmaev V, Manoharan A, Ramakrishna R. The potential role of curcumin in patients with monoclonal gammopathy of undefined significance--its effect on paraproteinemia and the urinary N-telopeptide of type I collagen bone turnover marker. Clin Cancer Res 2009; 15(18): 5917-22.
[http://dx.doi.org/10.1158/1078-0432.CCR-08-2217] [PMID: 19737963]

[65]   Durgaprasad S, Pai CG, Vasanthkumar , Alvres JF, Namitha S. A pilot study of the antioxidant effect of curcumin in tropical pancreatitis. Indian J Med Res 2005; 122(4): 315-8.
[PMID: 16394323]

[66]   Belcaro G, Cesarone MR, Dugall M, *et al.* Product-evaluation registry of Meriva®, a curcumin-phosphatidylcholine complex, for the complementary management of osteoarthritis. Panminerva Med 2010; 52(2) (Suppl. 1): 55-62.
[PMID: 20657536]

[67]   Belcaro G, Cesarone MR, Dugall M, *et al.* Efficacy and safety of Meriva®, a curcumin-phosphatidylcholine complex, during extended administration in osteoarthritis patients. Altern Med Rev 2010; 15(4): 337-44.
[PMID: 21194249]

[68]   Chandran B, Goel A. A randomized, pilot study to assess the efficacy and safety of curcumin in patients with active rheumatoid arthritis. Phytother Res 2012; 26(11): 1719-25.
[http://dx.doi.org/10.1002/ptr.4639] [PMID: 22407780]

[69]   Panahi Y, Sahebkar A, Amiri M, *et al.* Improvement of sulphur mustard-induced chronic pruritus, quality of life and antioxidant status by curcumin: results of a randomised, double-blind, placebo-controlled trial. Br J Nutr 2012; 108(7): 1272-9.
[http://dx.doi.org/10.1017/S0007114511006544] [PMID: 22099425]

[70]   Kurd SK, Smith N, VanVoorhees A, *et al.* Oral curcumin in the treatment of moderate to severe psoriasis vulgaris: A prospective clinical trial. J Am Acad Dermatol 2008; 58(4): 625-31.
[http://dx.doi.org/10.1016/j.jaad.2007.12.035] [PMID: 18249471]

[71]   Bahraini P, Rajabi M, Mansouri P, Sarafian G, Chalangari R, Azizian Z. Turmeric tonic as a treatment in scalp psoriasis: A randomized placebo-control clinical trial. J Cosmet Dermatol 2018; 17(3): 461-6.
[http://dx.doi.org/10.1111/jocd.12513] [PMID: 29607625]

[72]   Heng MC, Song MK, Harker J, Heng MK. Drug-induced suppression of phosphorylase kinase activity correlates with resolution of psoriasis as assessed by clinical, histological and immunohistochemical parameters. Br J Dermatol 2000; 143(5): 937-49.
[http://dx.doi.org/10.1046/j.1365-2133.2000.03767.x] [PMID: 11069500]

[73]   Antiga E, Bonciolini V, Volpi W, Del Bianco E, Caproni M. Oral curcumin (Meriva) is effective as an adjuvant treatment and is able to reduce IL-22 serum levels in patients with psoriasis vulgaris. BioMed Research International 2015; 2015.

[74]   Asawanonda P, Klahan SO. Tetrahydrocurcuminoid cream plus targeted narrowband UVB phototherapy for vitiligo: a preliminary randomized controlled study. Photomed Laser Surg 2010; 28(5): 679-84.
[http://dx.doi.org/10.1089/pho.2009.2637] [PMID: 20961233]

[75]   James JS. Curcumin: clinical trial finds no antiviral effect. AIDS Treat News 1996; (242): 1-2.
[PMID: 11363190]

[76]   Fadus MC, Lau C, Bikhchandani J, Lynch HT. Curcumin: An age-old anti-inflammatory and anti-neoplastic agent. J Tradit Complement Med 2016; 7(3): 339-46.
[http://dx.doi.org/10.1016/j.jtcme.2016.08.002] [PMID: 28725630]

[77]   Singletary K. Turmeric: Potential Health Benefits. Nutr Today 2020; 55(1): 45-56.
[http://dx.doi.org/10.1097/NT.0000000000000392]

[78]   Goel A, Kunnumakkara AB, Aggarwal BB. Curcumin as "Curecumin": from kitchen to clinic. Biochem Pharmacol 2008; 75(4): 787-809.
[http://dx.doi.org/10.1016/j.bcp.2007.08.016] [PMID: 17900536]

[79]   Rahmani AH, Alsahli MA, Aly SM, Khan MA, Aldebasi YH. Role of curcumin in disease prevention and treatment. Adv Biomed Res 2018; 7: 38.
[http://dx.doi.org/10.4103/abr.abr_147_16] [PMID: 29629341]

CHAPTER 5

Origanum majorana: The Fragrance of Health

Bhushan P. Pimple[*], **Amrita M. Kulkarni** and **Ruchita B. Bhor**

P. E. Society's Modern College of Pharmacy, Yamunanagar, Nigdi, Pune, India 411044

Abstract: *Origanum majorana* Linn. (*Majorana hortensis*) is an aromatic herb of Lamiaceae. The plant is native to Mediterranean and European parts, but can be cultivated easily in all tropical regions. The leaves and flowers are characterized by a pleasant aromatic odour that increases its scope for perfumery and food industries. Besides its culinary & perfumery importance, *O. majorana* has therapeutic relevance in the management of diabetes, hypertension, polycystic ovarian syndrome (PCOS), gastric ulcers, leukemia, breast adenocarcinoma, free radical scavenging, *etc*. The proposed chapter focuses on traditional uses, culinary and perfumery applications, recent advancements in phytochemistry and pharmacotherapeutics of *Origanum majorana*.

Keywords: Adenocarcinoma, Hyperglycemia, Hypertension, *Origanum majorana*, Sweet majorana.

INTRODUCTION

Traditional Claims [1 - 9]

1. Decoction of fresh aerial parts of *Origanum majorana* was consumed to relieve flatulence in Colombia.
2. *Origanum majorana* was used as a constituent in many herbal mixtures in Eastern Cuba for treating diabetes, catarrh, stomach pains and as a sedative.
3. Majorana is still used as a traditional herb for cough, stomach aches and as a carminative in Jordan.
4. *Origanum* spp. were used to produce sedation and for treating insomnia in Italy.
5. Infusion of majorana leaves is a traditional application for hypertension in Morocco.

---

[*] **Corresponding author Bhushan P. Pimple:** Department of Pharmacognosy, P.E. Society's Modern College of Pharmacy, Yamunanagar, Nigdi, Pune, Maharashtra, India 411 044; Tel: +91 2027661314/15; E-mail: bhushanppimple@rediffmail.com

Atta-ur-Rahman, M. Iqbal Choudhary & Sammer Yousuf (Eds.)

6. In Cyprus, leaves of *Origanum majorana* in the form of infusion or inhalation were used to treat diabetes, hypertension, diarrhoea, migraine, stomach ache, cough, dysmenorrhea, asthma, bronchitis.

7. In India, *Piper nigrum* and *Origanum* spp. were mixed to form a paste and applied overboils, ulcers, fire burns and cuts. It was used for menstrual complaints, cold and fever.

8. The traditional medicinal system in Germany includes *Origanum majorana* as an anti-fertility herb.

9. *Origanum* is one of the traditional herbs in Austrian medicine put into tea and externally used as an ointment (see Fig. **1**).

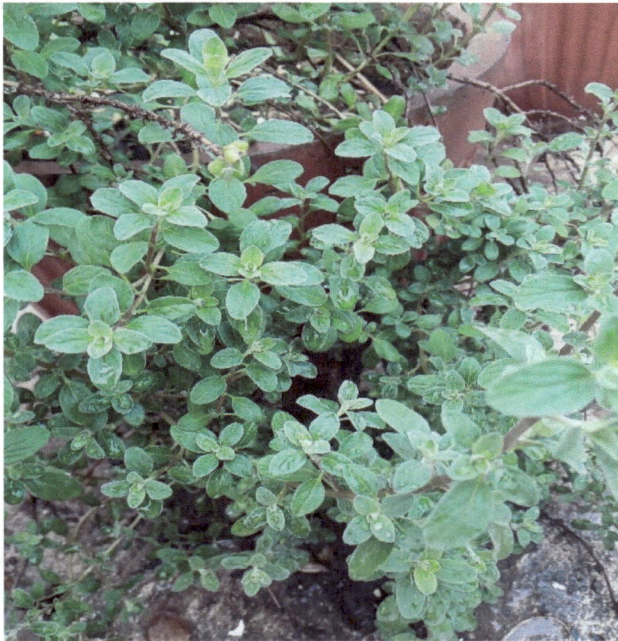

Fig. (1). Leaves of *Origanum majorana.*

Vernacular Names [10]

Hindi: *Marwa*

Bengali: *Murru*

Tamil: *Marru, Maruvu*

Kannada: *Maruga*

Malyalam: *Maruvanu*

Kumaun: *Bantulsi*

Deccan: *Murwa*

DRUG INTERACTIONS [11 - 14]

The details of the drug interaction of *Origanum majorana* with other plants are mentioned in **Table 1.**

Table 1. Drug interactions of *Origanum majorana* with other plants.

Combinations with *Origanum majorana*	Targets	Effects	Mechanism	References
Essential Oils of *Origanum compactum*, ***Origanum majorana***, *Thymus serphyllum*	*Escherichia coli, Staphylococcus aureus, Bacillus subtiltis*	Bactericidal effect (Death of the bacteria)	Impair the structure and functioning of the bacterial cell membrane.	[11]
Azadirachta indica, Ocimum sanctum, Withania somnifera and ***Origanum majorana***	DNA damage caused by alkylation (O^6-alkylguanines) on Human colon carcinoma cell lines HT29 and HCT116	DNA repair evident.	Upregulation of O^6-methylguanine DNA methyltransferase (MGMT), a protein which aids DNA repair corresponding to DNA damage.	[12]
Lemon balm, **Marjoram**, Oregano and Thyme	*Enterobacter* spp., *Listeria* spp., *Lactobacillus* spp., and *Pseudomonas* spp. in food model media based on lettuce, meat and milk	Antimicrobial effect	Presence of the hydroxyl group in the essential oils exhibited antimicrobial effect.	[13]
Essential oils of **Marjoram**, Rosemary and Basil	Free radical 2,2-diphenyl-1-picrylhydrazyl (DPPH)	Antioxidant activity	Free radical scavenging due to essential oil components.	[14]

PHYTOCHEMISTRY OF *ORIGANUM MAJORANA* [14 - 25]

The details of the phytochemistry of *Origanum majorana* are mentioned in Table **2.**

THERAPEUTIC USES [26 - 29]

- It is used to treat anxiety.
- It is used to treat diabetes.
- It can be used against convulsions and seizures.
- It has an insecticidal, nematocidal and molluscicidal activity.

Table 2. Phytoconstituents of *Origanum majorana*.

Chemical class of Phytoconstituent	Phytoconstituents	Significance of Phytoconstituents	References
Essential Oils	Carvacrol, thymol, terpinen-4-ol, cis sabinene hydrate, trans sabinene hydrate, p- cymene, γ-terpinene, α-thujene, camphene, sabinene, α- terpinol α- terpinene, bornyl acetate, linalool, α-pinene, α-terpineol iso-sylvestrene, β-pinene limonene, 1,8-cineole, 3- octanol, myrcene, β-phellandrene, linalyl acetate,	Essential oils from *Origanum majorana* exhibited potent antioxidant activity against DPPH radical. Linalool, α-terpineol and linalyl acetate were predicted to scavenge the DPPH radical. Carvacrol exhibited neuroprotective effects against peripheral neurodegeneration by inhibiting TRP melastatin M7 (TRPM7) receptor in Schwann cells, thereby protecting the demyelination of peripheral nerves.	[14 - 19]
Phenolic compounds: **1. Phenolic acids** **2. Phenolic glycosides**	Hydroxyquinone Vanillic acid, Gallic acid, Ferulic acid, Caffeic acid, p and m- hydroxybenzoic acid, coumaric acid, rosmarinic acid, chlorogenic acid, cryptochlorogenic, neochlorogenic acid. Syringic acid *trans*-2-Hydroxycinnamic acid, coumaric acid, cinnamic acid, lithospermic acid Arbutin, Methyl arbutin, Vitexin	Lee *et al.* studied the UV absorption, DPPH radial and Nitric oxide scavenging property, tyrosinase inhibition of phenolic compounds in *O.majorana,* the compounds possessed strong antioxidant, UV absorption, and tyrosinase inhibitory property and highlighted the importance in skincare products.	[17, 20, 21, 22]

(Table 2) cont.....

Chemical class of Phytoconstituent	Phytoconstituents	Significance of Phytoconstituents	References
Flavonoids	Amentoflavone, Apigenin, Quercetin, Luteolin, Coumarin, Rutin Hesperetin	Apigenin, Luteolin possess anti-inflammatory activity by inhibiting proinflammatory mediators cyclooxygenase, nitric oxide synthase.	[17, 20, 23]
Flavanones	naringenin narirutin O – rutinoside eriocitrin O – rutinoside hesperidin O – rutinoside		[24]
Flavones	Apigenein, Isorhoifolin, Luteolin, 5,6,3'-Trihydroxy-7,8,4'-trimethoxyflavone Baicalein	Baicalein inhibits α-glucosidase enzyme, thereby prohibiting the release of glucose from polysaccharides. Active against metabolic disorders like diabetes mellitus, metastatic cancers and HIV infection.	[20, 24, 25]
Flavonoid glycoside	Kaempferol-3-O-glucoside Quercetin-3-O-glucoside Narigenin-O-hexoside Apigenin-glucuronide Rutin Luteolin-7 β -O--glucuronide		[21]

GLOBAL AND INDIAN MARKET OF *ORIGANUM MAJORANA* [30, 31]

Import Data [30, 31]

Top Suppliers of *Origanum majorana* are France, Germany and United Kingdom, while others include Switzerland, Egypt and Spain.

Export of Marjoram Oil [30, 31]

Marjoram oil has been exported to Czech Republic, South Korea, United Kingdom, Thailand, Poland.

Toxicity of *Origanum Majorana* [21]

Origanum majorana can be toxic to the foetus due to its emmenagogue properties. It must be avoided during pregnancy and in lactating mothers.

PHARMACOLOGY [32 - 48]

Antioxidant Activity

Origanum majorana essential oil contains rosmarinic acid and carnosol, which exhibit strong antioxidant activity by scavenging hydroxyl radicals [32].

Jun *et al.* isolated and purified a phenolic compound T3b from methanol extract of *Origanum majorana*, it possessed *in-vitro* superoxide anion radical scavenging activity, stronger than other natural antioxidants. T3b prevented the 12--tetradecanolyphorbol-13-acetate (TPA)-induced O_2 generation and hydrogen peroxide formation in differentiated HL-60 cells (Human Leukemia cell line) [33].

Antimicrobial Activity

Phenolic compounds in the essential oil (Carvacrol, thymol, Terpinene) possess antimicrobial property due to their ability to destroy the cell membrane, electron transport, active transport and coagulation of cell contents in the bacteria [34].

Lower concentration of *O. majorana* essential oil was bacteriostatic and higher concentrations exhibited a bactericidal in food sausage preparation. Phenols in the essential oil disrupted the cell membrane of the Gram-positive bacteria than the Gram-negative bacteria [35].

Stamatis *et al.* studied the inhibitory action of *Origanum* spp. on *Helicobacter pylori*. 70% methanol extract of *Origanum majorana* inhibited the growth of *Helicobacter pylori*, proving its gastroprotective effects [36].

Antigenotoxic Effect

Hydroquinone (HQ) is genotoxic and induces micronuclei (MN), sister-chromatid exchange (SCE), and chromosomal aberrations. *Zizyphus jujuba* and *O. majorana* extracts showed protection against these clastogenic effects (chromosomal aberrations) of HQ in mice due to their pronounced antioxidant activity and ability to scavenge free radicals generated by HQ [37].

Antigenotoxic effect of essential oils of *Origanum majorana* was investigated against Prallethrin (insecticide) induced genotoxic damage in rat bone marrow cells. Genotoxicity led to chromosomal aberrations and micronuclei formation in the bone marrow cells, treatment with *Origanum majorana* essential oils reduced the chromosomal aberrations and micronuclei formation by scavenging genotoxicity inducing free radicals [38].

Anti-hyperglycaemic

Lemhadri *et al.* studied the hypoglycaemic activity of *Origanum* sp. in normal and streptozotocin (STZ) induced diabetic rats. The aqueous extract of the leaves exerted a potent anti-hyperglycaemic activity in diabetic rats. The hypoglycaemic effect is attributed to the decreased hepatic glucose production and increased peripheral glucose uptake without affecting insulin secretion [39].

Anti-depressant

Maleki *et al.* evaluated the anti- depressant activity of *Origanum majorana* essential oil in mice. Antidepressant activity involved the D1, D2, 5-HT1A, 5-HT2A, a1 and a2 receptors (Dopamine, serotonin and adrenergic), thus pre-treatment with respective blockers prevented the antidepressant effects. However, antidepressants and marjoram essential oil exhibited synergism against depression in mice [40].

Anti- neurodegenerative Effect

Rosmarinic acid in the aqueous extract of *O.majorana* possessed anti-neurodegenerative activity, due to its antioxidant and anti-neurodegenerative activities by acetylcholinesterase inhibition [41].

Anti-proliferative Activity

The anti- proliferative activity of *Origanum majorana* was determined on the human lymphoblastic leukemia cell line. *O. majorana* extracts stimulated apoptosis, due to an up-regulation of p53 protein levels and down-regulation of Bcl-2alpha [42].

Essential oils of *Origanum majorana* proved to be cytotoxic and inhibited cellular growth of Human colorectal cancer cell lines (HT-9 cell lines). Essential oils induced autophagy and caspase-dependent cleavage of p70S6K (a protein overexpressed in colon cancer cells) induced apoptosis in HT-9 cancer cell lines [43].

Anti-spasmodic and Myorelaxant Activity

The anti-spasmodic activity of organic fractions from *Origanum majorana* was studied on rabbit jejunum. Amongst all of those, dichloromethane fraction exhibited remarkable anti-spasmodic activity and myorelaxant effect on rabbit intestinal spontaneous contractions [44].

Anti-urolithic Activity (Inhibition of Kidney Stones)

Origanum spp. can be used to treat urolithiasis due to its interference with Calcium oxalate crystal growth and aggregation; therefore, it seems a possible therapeutic strategy for the prevention of recurrent stone disease. It inhibits calcium oxalate crystal nucleation and aggregation and exhibited diuretic activity [45].

Cardioprotective Activity

Protective effects against hematological changes and cardiotoxicity due to isoproterenol in albino rats were observed when aqueous extract and leaf powder of *O. majorana* were administered. Isoproterenol administration led to erythrocytosis with an increase in Hb content, granulocytosis, thrombocytosis and shortened clotting time, increased the relative heart weight (cardiac hypertrophy) and leakage of heart enzymes. High doses of aqueous extract and leaf powder strengthened the antioxidant defence system of heart tissues [46].

Anti-ulcerogenic Activity

Marjoram ethanol extract exhibited gastroprotective effects against peptic ulcers and gastric damage in the rat model. Administration of marjoram extract decreased the gastric mucosal damage, intensity and severity of ulcers induced by indomethacin. Decreased volume and acidity of gastric secretions were evident. Extract replenished the gastric wall mucus and decreased the level of Malondialdehyde (MDA) in stomach tissue. Flavonoids, tannins, sterols possess gastroprotective effects [47].

Modulation of Polycystic Ovarian Syndrome (PCOS)

Marjoram tea modulated insulin sensitivity and regulated androgen levels in women diagnosed with PCOS. Marjoram can be used to regulate the menstrual cycle [48].

VETERINARY APPLICATIONS [49 - 53]

1. Administration of origanum oil enhanced milk quality (fat and protein) in China Holstein Cows.
2. *Origanum* spp. have been used for respiratory, liver, kidney, gall, urinary tract disorders and as an anthelmintic in Azerbaijan.
3. The essential oil of *O. majorana* is used against pathogenic fungi in veterinary medicine.
4. *Origanum majorana* at a concentration of 200–500 µL/L induced anaesthesia in 200-800 seconds in fish.
5. The addition of essential oils of *Origanum vulgare* and *Citrus* spp. in the diet of sheep inhibited the occurrence and intensity of coccidian infection, promoted lamb growth and higher meat quality.

CONSENT FOR PUBLICATION

Not applicable.

CONFLICT OF INTEREST

The authors confirm that there is no conflict of interest.

ACKNOWLEDGEMENTS

None Declared.

REFERENCES

[1]   Gómez-Estrada H, Díaz-Castillo F, Franco-Ospina L, *et al.* Folk medicine in the northern coast of Colombia: an overview. J Ethnobiol Ethnomed 2011; 7(1): 27.
[http://dx.doi.org/10.1186/1746-4269-7-27] [PMID: 21939522]

[2]   Cano JH, Volpato G. Herbal mixtures in the traditional medicine of eastern Cuba. J Ethnopharmacol 2004; 90(2-3): 293-316.
[http://dx.doi.org/10.1016/j.jep.2003.10.012] [PMID: 15013195]

[3]   Hudaib M, Mohammad M, Bustanji Y, *et al.* Ethnopharmacological survey of medicinal plants in Jordan, Mujib Nature Reserve and surrounding area. J Ethnopharmacol 2008; 120(1): 63-71.
[http://dx.doi.org/10.1016/j.jep.2008.07.031] [PMID: 18760342]

[4]   Scherrer AM, Motti R, Weckerle CS. Traditional plant use in the areas of monte vesole and ascea, cilento national park (Campania, Southern Italy). J Ethnopharmacol 2005; 97(1): 129-43.
[http://dx.doi.org/10.1016/j.jep.2004.11.002] [PMID: 15652287]

[5]   Tahraoui A, El-Hilaly J, Israili ZH, Lyoussi B. Ethnopharmacological survey of plants used in the traditional treatment of hypertension and diabetes in south-eastern Morocco (Errachidia province). J Ethnopharmacol 2007; 110(1): 105-17.
[http://dx.doi.org/10.1016/j.jep.2006.09.011] [PMID: 17052873]

[6]   Karousou R, Deirmentzoglou S. The herbal market of Cyprus: traditional links and cultural exchanges. J Ethnopharmacol 2011; 133(1): 191-203.
[http://dx.doi.org/10.1016/j.jep.2010.09.034] [PMID: 20920568]

[7]   Sharma PK, Chauhan NS, Lal B. Observations on the traditional phytotherapy among the inhabitants of Parvati valley in western Himalaya, India. J Ethnopharmacol 2004; 92(2-3): 167-76.
[http://dx.doi.org/10.1016/j.jep.2003.12.018] [PMID: 15137998]

[8]   Maurya R, Srivastava S, Kulshreshta DK, Gupta CM. Traditional remedies for fertility regulation. Curr Med Chem 2004; 11(11): 1431-50.
[http://dx.doi.org/10.2174/0929867043365215] [PMID: 15180576]

[9]   Vogl S, Picker P, Mihaly-Bison J, *et al.* Ethnopharmacological *in vitro* studies on Austria's folk medicine--an unexplored lore *in vitro* anti-inflammatory activities of 71 Austrian traditional herbal drugs. J Ethnopharmacol 2013; 149(3): 750-71.
[http://dx.doi.org/10.1016/j.jep.2013.06.007] [PMID: 23770053]

[10]   Vasudeva N, Prerna G. *Origanum majorana* L-Phyto-pharmacological review. Indian J Nat Prod Resour 2015; 6(4): 261-7.

[11]   Ouedrhiri W, Balouiri M, Bouhdid S, *et al.* Mixture design of *Origanum compactum*, *Origanum majorana* and *Thymus serphyllum* essential oils: optimization of their antibacterial effect. Ind Crops Prod 2016; 89: 1-9.

[12]   Niture SK, Rao US, Srivenugopal KS. Chemopreventative strategies targeting the MGMT repair protein: augmented expression in human lymphocytes and tumor cells by ethanolic and aqueous extracts of several Indian medicinal plants. Int J Oncol 2006; 29(5): 1269-78.
[PMID: 17016661]

[13]   Gutierrez J, Barry-Ryan C, Bourke P. Antimicrobial activity of plant essential oils using food model media: efficacy, synergistic potential and interactions with food components. Food Microbiol 2009; 26(2): 142-50.
[PMID: 19171255]

[14]   Baj T, Baryluk A, Sieniawska E. Application of mixture design for optimum antioxidant activity of mixtures of essential oils from *Ocimum basilicum* L., *Origanum majorana* L. and *Rosmarinus officinalis* L. Ind Crops Prod 2018; 115: 52-61.
[http://dx.doi.org/10.1016/j.indcrop.2018.02.006]

[15]   Vokou D, Kokkini S, Bessiere JM. Geographic variation of Greek oregano (*Origanum vulgare* ssp. hirtum) essential oils. Biochem Syst Ecol 1993; 21(2): 287-95.
[http://dx.doi.org/10.1016/0305-1978(93)90047-U]

[16]   Vera RR, Chane-Ming J. Chemical composition of the essential oil of marjoram (*Origanum majorana* L.) from Reunion Island. Food Chem 1999; 66(2): 143-5.
[http://dx.doi.org/10.1016/S0308-8146(98)00018-1]

[17]   Sellami IH, Maamouri E, Chahed T, Wannes WA, Kchouk ME, Marzouk B. Effect of growth stage on the content and composition of the essential oil and phenolic fraction of sweet marjoram (*Origanum majorana* L.). Ind Crops Prod 2009; 30(3): 395-402.
[http://dx.doi.org/10.1016/j.indcrop.2009.07.010]

[18]   Amor G, Caputo L, La Storia A, De Feo V, Mauriello G, Fechtali T. Chemical composition and antimicrobial activity of artemisia herba-alba and *Origanum majorana* essential oils from Morocco. Molecules 2019; 24(22): 4021.
[http://dx.doi.org/10.3390/molecules24224021] [PMID: 31698834]

[19] Chun SS, Vattem DA, Lin YT, Shetty K. Phenolic antioxidants from clonal oregano (*Origanum vulgare*) with antimicrobial activity against *Helicobacter pylori*. Process Biochem 2005; 40(2): 809-16.

[20] Erenler R, Sen O, Aksit H, *et al*. Isolation and identification of chemical constituents from *Origanum majorana* and investigation of antiproliferative and antioxidant activities. J Sci Food Agric 2016; 96(3): 822-36.
[PMID: 25721137]

[21] Bina F, Rahimi R. Sweet marjoram: a review of ethnopharmacology, phytochemistry, and biological activities. J Evid Based Complementary Altern Med 2017; 22(1): 175-85.
[http://dx.doi.org/10.1177/2156587216650793] [PMID: 27231340]

[22] Lee CJ, Chen LG, Chang TL, Ke WM, *et al*. The correlation between skin-care effects and phytochemical contents in Lamiaceae plants. Food Chem 2011; 124(3): 833-41.
[http://dx.doi.org/10.1016/j.foodchem.2010.07.003]

[23] Mueller M, Lukas B, Novak J, Simoncini T, Genazzani AR, Jungbauer A. Oregano: a source for peroxisome proliferator-activated receptor γ antagonists. J Agric Food Chem 2008; 56(24): 11621-30.
[http://dx.doi.org/10.1021/jf802298w] [PMID: 19053389]

[24] Fecka I, Turek S. Determination of polyphenolic compounds in commercial herbal drugs and spices from Lamiaceae: thyme, wild thyme and sweet marjoram by chromatographic techniques. Food Chem 2008; 108(3): 1039-53.
[http://dx.doi.org/10.1016/j.foodchem.2007.11.035] [PMID: 26065769]

[25] de Melo EB, da Silveira Gomes A, Carvalho I. α-and β-Glucosidase inhibitors: chemical structure and biological activity. Tetrahedron 2006; 62(44): 10277-302.
[http://dx.doi.org/10.1016/j.tet.2006.08.055]

[26] Rezaie A, Mousavi G, Nazeri M, *et al*. Comparative study of sedative, pre-anesthetic and anti-anxiety effect of *Origanum majorana* extract with diazepam on rats. Res J Biol Sci 2011; 6(11): 611-4.
[http://dx.doi.org/10.3923/rjbsci.2011.611.614]

[27] Perez Gutierrez RM. Inhibition of advanced glycation end-product formation by *Origanum majorana* L. *in vitro* and in streptozotocin-induced diabetic rats. Evid Based Complementary Altern Med 2012; 2012(1): 598638.

[28] Deshmane DN, Gadgoli CH, Halade GV. Anticonvulsant effect of *Origanum majorana* L. Pharmacologyonline 2007; 1: 64-78.

[29] Tripathy B, Satyanarayana S, Khan KA, Raja K. An updated review on traditional uses, taxonomy, phytochemistry, pharmacology and toxicology of *Origanum majorana*. Int J Pharma Res Health Sci 2017; 5: 1717-23.

[30] https://www.zauba.com/[home page on Internet] Zauba Technologies Pvt Ltd 2018. Available from: https://www.zauba.com/import-marjoram/hs-code-33012990-hs-code.html

[31] https://www.zauba.com/[home page on Internet] Zauba Technologies Pvt Ltd 2018. Available from: https://www.zauba.com/export-marjoram-hs-code.html

[32] Brewer MS. Natural antioxidants: sources, compounds, mechanisms of action, and potential applications. Compr Rev Food Sci Food Saf 2011; 10(4): 221-47.
[http://dx.doi.org/10.1111/j.1541-4337.2011.00156.x]

[33] Jun WJ, Han BK, Yu KW, *et al*. Antioxidant effects of *Origanum majorana* L. on superoxide anion radicals. Food Chem 2001; 75(4): 439-44.
[http://dx.doi.org/10.1016/S0308-8146(01)00233-3]

[34] Burt S. Essential oils: their antibacterial properties and potential applications in foods--a review. Int J Food Microbiol 2004; 94(3): 223-53.
[http://dx.doi.org/10.1016/j.ijfoodmicro.2004.03.022] [PMID: 15246235]

[35]   Busatta C, Vidal RS, Popiolski AS, *et al.* Application of *Origanum majorana* L. essential oil as an antimicrobial agent in sausage. Food Microbiol 2008; 25(1): 207-11.
[http://dx.doi.org/10.1016/j.fm.2007.07.003] [PMID: 17993397]

[36]   Stamatis G, Kyriazopoulos P, Golegou S, Basayiannis A, Skaltsas S, Skaltsa H. *in vitro* anti-*Helicobacter pylori* activity of Greek herbal medicines. J Ethnopharmacol 2003; 88(2-3): 175-9.
[http://dx.doi.org/10.1016/S0378-8741(03)00217-4] [PMID: 12963139]

[37]   Ghaly IS, Said A, Abdel-Wahhab MA. *Zizyphus jujuba* and *Origanum majorana* extracts protect against hydroquinone-induced clastogenicity. Environ Toxicol Pharmacol 2008; 25(1): 10-9.
[http://dx.doi.org/10.1016/j.etap.2007.07.002] [PMID: 21783830]

[38]   Mossa AT, Refaie AA, Ramadan A, Bouajila J. Antimutagenic effect of *Origanum majorana* L. essential oil against prallethrin-induced genotoxic damage in rat bone marrow cells. J Med Food 2013; 16(12): 1101-7.
[http://dx.doi.org/10.1089/jmf.2013.0006] [PMID: 24195751]

[39]   Lemhadri A, Zeggwagh NA, Maghrani M, Jouad H, Eddouks M. Anti-hyperglycaemic activity of the aqueous extract of *Origanum vulgare* growing wild in Tafilalet region. J Ethnopharmacol 2004; 92(2-3): 251-6.
[http://dx.doi.org/10.1016/j.jep.2004.02.026] [PMID: 15138008]

[40]   Abbasi-Maleki S, Kadkhoda Z, Taghizad-Farid R. The antidepressant-like effects of *Origanum majorana* essential oil on mice through monoaminergic modulation using the forced swimming test. J Tradit Complement Med 2019; 10(4): 327-5.
[http://dx.doi.org/10.1016/j.jtcme.2019.01.003]

[41]   Duletić-Laušević S, Aradski AA, Kolarević S, *et al.* Antineurodegenerative, antioxidant and antibacterial activities and phenolic components of *Origanum majorana* L.(Lamiaceae) extracts. J Appl Bot Food Qual 2018; 91: 126-34.

[42]   Abdel-Massih RM, Fares R, Bazzi S, El-Chami N, Baydoun E. The apoptotic and anti-proliferative activity of *Origanum majorana* extracts on human leukemic cell line. Leuk Res 2010; 34(8): 1052-6.
[http://dx.doi.org/10.1016/j.leukres.2009.09.018] [PMID: 19853912]

[43]   Athamneh K, Alneyadi A, Alsamri H, *et al. Origanum majorana* essential oil triggers p38 mapk-mediated protective autophagy, apoptosis, and caspase-dependent cleavage of P70S6K in colorectal cancer cells. Biomolecules 2020; 10(3): 412.
[http://dx.doi.org/10.3390/biom10030412] [PMID: 32155920]

[44]   Makrane H, Aziz M, Berrabah M, *et al.* Myorelaxant Activity of essential oil from *Origanum majorana* L. on rat and rabbit. J Ethnopharmacol 2019; 228: 40-9.
[http://dx.doi.org/10.1016/j.jep.2018.08.036] [PMID: 30205180]

[45]   Khan A, Bashir S, Khan SR, Gilani AH. Antiurolithic activity of *Origanum vulgare* is mediated through multiple pathways. BMC Complement Altern Med 2011; 11(1): 96.
[PMID: 22004514]

[46]   Ramadan G, El-Beih NM, Arafa NM, Zahra MM. Preventive effects of Egyptian sweet marjoram (*Origanum majorana* L.) leaves on haematological changes and cardiotoxicity in isoproterenol-treated albino rats. Cardiovasc Toxicol 2013; 13(2): 100-9.
[PMID: 23054890]

[47]   Al-Howiriny T, Alsheikh A, Alqasoumi S, Al-Yahya M, ElTahir K, Rafatullah S. Protective Effect of *Origanum majorana* L. 'Marjoram' on various models of gastric mucosal injury in rats. Am J Chin Med 2009; 37(3): 531-45.
[http://dx.doi.org/10.1142/S0192415X0900703X] [PMID: 19606513]

[48]   Haj-Husein I, Tukan S, Alkazaleh F. The effect of marjoram (*Origanum majorana*) tea on the hormonal profile of women with polycystic ovary syndrome: a randomised controlled pilot study. J Hum Nutr Diet 2016; 29(1): 105-11.

[PMID: 25662759]

[49]   Liguo Y, Hengmin T, Jianzhong S. Study on application of oil origanum and flavomycin in dairy productsuction. Feed Industry 2004; p. 1. J

[50]   Agayeva Agayeva EZ, Ibadullayeva SJ, Asgerov AA, Isayeva GA. Analysis of plants in veterinary research of Azerbaycan on ethnobotanical materials. American Journal of Research Communication 2013; 1(4): 51-9.

[51]   Waller SB, Cleff MB, Serra EF, *et al.* Plants from Lamiaceae family as source of antifungal molecules in humane and veterinary medicine. Microb Pathog 2017; 104: 232-7.
[http://dx.doi.org/10.1016/j.micpath.2017.01.050] [PMID: 28131955]

[52]   Hoseini SM, Taheri Mirghaed A, Yousefi M. Application of herbal anaesthetics in aquaculture. Rev Aquacult 2018; 11(3): 550-64.

[53]   Dudko P, Junkuszew A, Bojar W, *et al.* Effect of dietary supplementation with preparation comprising the blend of essential oil from *Origanum vulgare* (Lamiaceae) and Citrus spp.(citraceae) on coccidia invasion and lamb growth. Ital J Anim Sci 2018; 17(1): 57-65.
[http://dx.doi.org/10.1080/1828051X.2017.1346965]

CHAPTER 6

Black Pepper (*Piper nigrum* L.): The King of Spices

Priyanka Soni[*], **Vishal Soni** and **Naveen Kumar Choudhary**

Department of Pharmacognosy, B.R. Nahata College of Pharmacy, Mandsaur, M.P., India

Abstract: *Piper nigrum* (family Piperaceae) is a valuable medicinal plant. Black pepper is one of the important spices, rich in aromatic and medicinal components along with an appreciable level of several other functional components having health-promoting properties. It contains major pungent alkaloid. Many investigators have isolated different types of compounds, *i.e.* Phenolics, flavonoids, alkaloids, amides and steroids, lignans, neo-lignans, terpenes and many other compounds. Some of the compounds are Brachyamide B, Dihydropipericide(2E,4E)-N-Eicosadieno-l-pereridine, N-trans-Feruloyltyramine, N-Formyl piperidine, (2E,4E)-N-isobuty ldecadienamid, isobutyl-eicosadienamide, Tricholein, Trichostachine, isobutyl-eicosatrienamide, Isobutyl-octadienamide, Piperamide, Piperamine, Piperettine, Pipericide, Piperine, Piperolein B, Sarmentine, Sarmentosine, Retrofractamide A. Black pepper is used as a medicinal agent, a preservative, and in perfumery. Whole Peppercorn of *Piper nigrum* or its active components is being used in different types of foods and as medicine. Piperine (1-peperoyl piperidine) is known to possess many interesting pharmacological actions such as antihypertensive and antiplatelets, antioxidant, antitumor, antiasthmatics, antipyretic, analgesic, anti-inflammatory, anti-diarrheal, antispasmodic, anxiolytic, antidepressants, hepato-protective, immuno-modulatory, antibacterial, antifungal, anti-thyroids, antiapoptotic, anti-metastatic, antimutagenic, anti-spermatogenic, anti-Colon toxin, insecticidal and larvicidal activities, *etc*. Piperine has been found to enhance the therapeutic efficacy of many drugs, vaccines and nutrients by increasing oral bioavailability and by inhibiting various metabolizing enzymes. It is also known to enhance cognitive action and fertility. Piperine is also found to stimulate the pancreatic and intestinal enzymes which aid in digestion. Many therapeutic activities of this spice are attributed to the presence of piperine apart from other chemical constituents. *Piper nigrum* is also used as a flavoring agent. Recently, many studies have shown anticancer activities of piperine, a pungent alkaloid found in black pepper and some other Piper species. The collected preclinical data can be useful in the design of future researches especially clinical trials with piperine. It is, therefore, concluded that black pepper and its bioactive compound, piperine exhibit wide spectrum therapeutic potential and have also emerged as an excellent adjuvant to enhance the therapeutic efficacy of the concurrently administered drugs and nutrients.

[*] **Corresponding author Priyanka Soni**: B.R. Nahata College of Pharmacy, Mandsaur, M.P., India; Tel: 9993346486; E-mail: soni_priyanka21@rediffmail.com

Atta-ur-Rahman, M. Iqbal Choudhary & Sammer Yousuf (Eds.)

Keywords: Black Pepper, Expectorant, Flavonoids, King of Spices, Medicinal agent, *Piper nigrum* L, Piperaceae, Piperine (1-peperoyl piperidine), pungent alkaloid.

INTRODUCTION

Piper nigrum is also known as "The King of spices" as it is the most commonly used spice in the world and also valued for its medicinal properties. *Piper nigrum* L. belongs to the piperaceae family. The genus Piper has more than 1000 species but frequently known are *Piper nigrum*, *Piper longum* and *Piper betle*. *Piper nigrum* is a perennial shrub grown in many tropical regions such as Brazil, Indonesia, Malaysia, Vietnam, and Southern India. In India, it is well grown in Western Ghats of Kerala, where it grows wild in the mountains. It is known by different local names such as Kali Mirch in Urdu and Hindi, Pippali in Sanskrit, Milagu in Tamil and Peppercorn, White pepper, Green pepper, *Black pepper*, Madagascar pepper in English [1, 2].

Black pepper is used as spice as well as medicine, preservative and biocontrol agent. According to various literature, it was traditionally used as gastroprotective, antiseptic, antimicrobial, antioxidant, anti-inflammatory, gastro-protective and antidepressant, antiseptic, antispasmodic, aromatic, analgesic, anti-toxicant, aphrodisiac, antipyretic, anti-rheumatic, anti-diabetic, diuretic, flavor, spirit, dyspepsia, to increase salivary secretion and promote digestion, as CNS stimulant, throat ache reliever, cold cure, germicidal, blood purifier, antibacterial, for religious value, anti-cancer, pungent, in kitchen curries, cough curing, carminative, insecticide, *etc.* Externally, it is used as a rubefacient and as a local applicator to relax the sore throat and some skin disorders [3 - 6].

The chief constituent of *Black pepper* is known as piperine, due to which *Black pepper* has diverse pharmacological activity. Piperine was discovered in 1819 by Hans Christian. The pharmacological activities of piperine include antihypertensive and antiplatelets, antioxidant, antitumor, antiasthmatics, antipyretic, analgesic, anti-inflammatory, anti-diarrheal, antispasmodic, anxio-lytic, antidepressants, hepato-protective, immunomodulatory, antibacterial, antifungal, anti-thyroids, antiapoptotic, anti-metastatic, antimutagenic, anti-spermatogenic, anti-colon toxin, insecticidal and larvicidal activities, *etc.* It was also reported that piperine has the potential to increase the therapeutic efficacy of many drugs, vaccines and nutrients by increasing oral bioavailability and inhibiting various metabolizing enzymes. Piperine also has the potential to minimize different mutations like ethyl carbamate induced mutation in Drosophila. While compared to mutation, *Black pepper* also reduced tumor formation in mice such as Ehrlich ascites tumor and Dolton's lymphoma cells [7, 8].

In the recent past, different articles have been published having therapeutic potentials of *Piper nigrum*, its extracts, or its chief chemical constituent "piperine". So, in the current review, it has been aimed to provide updated literature on recent pharmacognostic, phytochemical and pharmacological activities of *Piper nigrum* L.

PHARMACOGNOSTIC CHARACTERISTIC OF *BLACK PEPPER* PLANT

It is a flowering woody perennial climbing vine that belongs to the Piperaceae family. Pepper plants easily grow in the shade of supporting trees, trellises, or poles up to a maximum height of 3- 4 meters and the roots may come out from leaf nodes if the vine touches the ground. The plants have a heart shape alternate leaves being typically 5-10 cm in length and 3-6 cm across, with 5 to 7 prominent palmate veins. The flowers are small, monoecious with separate male and female flowers but may be polygamous containing both male and female flowers. The small flowers are born on pendulous spikes at the leaf nodes that are nearly as long as the leaves. The length of spikes goes up to 7-15 cm. The *Black pepper*'s fruits are small (3 to 4 mm in diameter) called a drupe and the dried unripe fruits of *Piper nigrum* are known as a peppercorn. The fully mature fruits are dark red and approximately 5 mm in diameter. Its fruit contains a single seed. The plants bear fruits from 4th or 5th year and continue to bear fruits up to seven years. A single stem contains 20-30 spikes of fruits. The collected spikes are sun-dried to separate the peppercorns from the spikes. The fresh harvested unripe green fruits may be freeze-dried to make green pepper. Whereas, the fresh harvested unripe green fruits may be sun-dried to make *Black pepper*. The red skin of the ripen fruits is removed and the stony seeds are sun-dried to make white pepper [9].

TAXONOMICAL CLASSIFICATION OF *PIPER NIGRUM*

Kingdom: Plantae

Subkingdom: Tracheobionta

Superdivision: Spermatophyta

Division: Magnoliophyta

Class: Magnoliopsida

Sub class: Magnoliidae

Order: Piperales

Family: Piperaceae

Genus: Piper

Species: *nigrum L.*

The result of morphology and microscopic characteristics of powdered *Black pepper* was reported by Shaheen N. *et al.* (2019). The powder was brownish to black, having an aromatic odor with a pungent taste. The powder microscopic study indicated the presence of Lignified endocarp cells, oil cells, Hypodermal parenchyma with stone cells, Pigmented epicarp, Perisperm with starch granules, Testa with reddish-brown pigments, stone cells, Mesocarp cells, Cluster of calcium oxalates, Pitted fiber, Fibrous sclereids, Annular vessel, Sclereids, Rectangular vessels, Parenchyma layer with oil cells, Starch granules, Covering trichomes with stomata, and Pigmented pericarp with crystal calcium oxalates [10] (Fig. **1**).

PHARMACOLOGICAL ACTIVITIES OF BLACK PEPPER

Antioxidant Activity

Herbs and plant products are widely used to scavenge free radicals generated in the body due to various activities. Many studies have been conducted for the evaluation of the antioxidant activity of *Piper nigrum*. Ilhami G. (2005) confirmed the strong antioxidant activity of 75 µg/ml concentration of Aqueous extract and Ethanolic extract which showed 95.5% and 93.3% antioxidant activity respectively against 1,1-Diphenyl-2-picrylhydrazyl (DPPH) free radical scavenging, superoxide anion radical scavenging, hydrogen peroxide scavenging, and metal chelating activities. Total phenolic content was also determined in 1 mg Aqueous and Ethanolic extract using FolinCiocalteu method and it was 54.3 and 42.8 µg gallic acid equivalent of phenols, respectively [11]. Ethanolic extract of *Piper nigrum* showed high antioxidant activity with 74.61±0.02% inhibition against DPPH with IC_{50} values 14.15±0.02 µg/mg, respectively. Here, IC_{50} is defined as the concentration of substrate required to scavenge 50% of DPPH [12]. The various activities show that *Piper nigrum* has good potential to scavenge free radicals and delay the aging process. As reported, it has antioxidant activity due to the presence of flavonoids and phenolic contents [13].

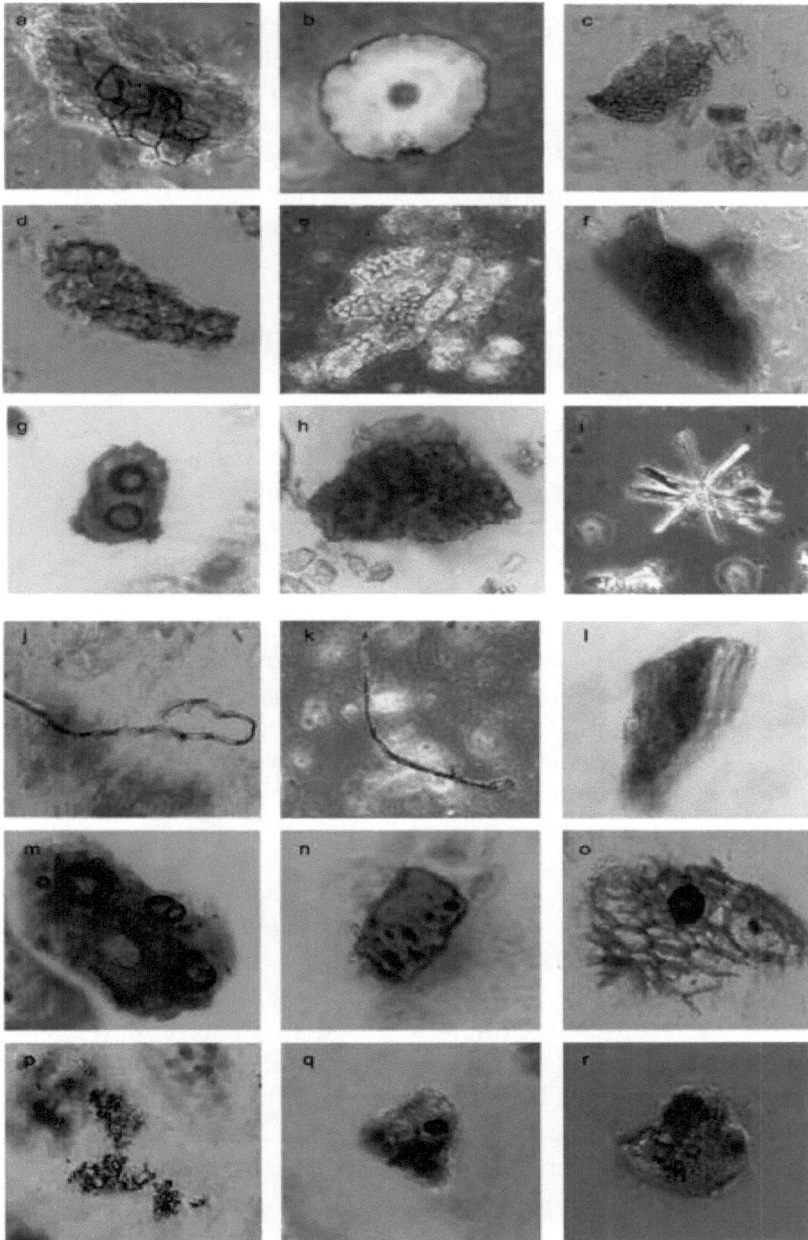

Fig. (1). The result of morphology and microscopic characteristics of powedered *Black pepper*.

Antimicrobial Activity

According to WHO, 50% of death or mortality worldwide is due to microbial infectious diseases [14]. Antimicrobial agents kill or inhibit microbes and bacteria. Many plants have been used as antimicrobial agents since ancient times. In the late 20th century, synthetic antibiotics were used to kill microbes but they acquire resistance against antibiotics and antimicrobial agents. So, in the last few years, again the antimicrobial activity has been investigated in plants and plant-derived products. Plants and plant-derived products also acquire resistance but it seems less due to the presence of a variety of chemical entities in a single plant. In literature, the *Black pepper* has been extensively studied for its antibacterial properties.

Abdallah *et al.* (2018) described the significant antimicrobial activity of *Black pepper* extracts (Ethanolic, methanolic, Aqueous) against major gram-negative and gram-positive strains by using the following antibacterial method, *i.e.* cup-plate method, disc diffusion method, micro-dilution method, or minimum inhibitory concentration. The study was performed on 6 Gram-Negative *Escherichia coli, Klebsiella pneumoniae, Salmonella typhi, Pseudomonas aeruginosa, Salmonella typhimurium,* and 7 Gram-Positive: *Staphylococcus aureus, Staphylococcus epidermidis, Enterococcus faecalis, Bacillus cereus, Bacillus subtilis, Bacillus megaterium, Streptococcus faecalis* bacteria. Ethanolic extract showed the highest inhibition against gram-negative (*Escherichia coli*) and gram-negative (*Staphylococcus aureus*) bacteria with 36 mm and 38 mm inhibition, respectively, in well diffusion method, whereas no activity was noticed with the methanolic extract [15].

In a study, the antibacterial mechanism was elucidated by analyzing cell morphology, respiratory metabolism, pyruvic acid content, and ATP levels of the target bacteria against *Escherichia coli* and *Staphylococcus aureus* using Chloroform extract of *Black pepper*. The Scanning electron microscope results showed that the bacterial cells exhibited adhesion, fracture, and accumulation. The antibacterial components of pepper restrained cellular respiration by disrupting the TCA pathway. The accumulation of pyruvic acid and the reduction of ATP proved that extract can change cell membrane permeability, destroy bacterial respiratory metabolism, and ultimately lead to pyknosis and death [16].

Antibacterial activity of *Black pepper* was also proved against *Streptococcus* mutants isolated from patients with tooth decay and inflammation of the teeth and *Escherichia coli* isolated from patients with diarrhea, by using the agar well diffusion method and microtiter plate method. The results revealed that the maximum inhibition region was 29 mm against *Streptococcus* mutants and minimum against *E. coli, i.e.* 8 mm [17].

Antidiarrheal Activity

Shaw Kumar PB *et al.* (2012) evaluated aqueous *Black pepper* extract for its anti-diarrheal, anti-motility, and anti-secretory activity using castor oil and magnesium sulphate-induced diarrhea, charcoal meal test and castor oil-induced intestinal secretions, respectively. They concluded that *Black pepper* has significant and dose-dependent anti-diarrheal activity due to its anti-motility and anti-secretory activity. The carbohydrates and alkaloids present are responsible for the anti-motility and anti-secretory activity [18]. Furthermore, it was also established that *Piper nigrum* has anti-diarrheal activity due to its involvement in the nitric oxide pathway and potassium channel blockage and opening [19].

In-vitro and *in-vivo* assay of *Black pepper* also revealed anti-secretory and antidiarrheal activity due to spasmodic (cholinergic) and antispasmodic (opioid agonist and Ca^{2+} antagonist) effects [20].

Analgesic, Anti-inflammatory and Antipyretic Activity

Several studies have revealed that *Piper nigrum* has potent analgesic and anti-inflammatory activity. Piperine, the chief constituent of *Black pepper*, Ethanolic, and Hexane extract of *Black pepper* was evaluated for analgesic activity using the tail immersion method, analgesic meter, hot plate and, acetic acid-induced writhing test. The results revealed that piperine, hexane, and ethanol extracts showed significant analgesic, anti-inflammatory activity with passage of time and maximum effect was achieved after 60 and 120 min [21].

Wnaga B *et al.* (2017) reported that the dichloromethane extract of *Piper nigrum* exhibited good anti-inflammatory activity in rats having cerebral ischemia by suppressing the production of Interleukin-1, Interleukin-6 and, TNF-α. In contrast, the extract also showed activity against permanent middle cerebral artery occlusion (PMCAO) injury by reducing free radicals evaluated *via* the Superoxide dismutase free radical suppression method [22]. Isolated piperine was evaluated for *in-vitro* anti-inflammatory activity using interleukin-1β (IL1β) stimulated fibroblast-like synoviocytes derived from rheumatoid arthritis patient and the results reported that piperine inhibited the release of IL1β and decreased the production of Prostaglandin E_2 in a dose-dependent manner. The *in-vivo* nociceptive and antiarthritic activities were evaluated *via* carrageenan-induced paw inflammation and arthritis with a dose of 20 and 100 mg/kg/day for 8 days; here results revealed significantly reduced nociceptive and arthritic symptoms [23].

The antipyretic and ulcerogenic effects of piperine were evaluated and it was found that piperine has significant antipyretic activity without ulcerogenic effect [24].

Anticonvulsant Activity

The anticonvulsant effect of piperine was evaluated using acetic acid-induced writhing, tail-flick assay, pentylenetetrazol (PTZ)- and picrotoxin (PIC)-induced seizures models. 30, 50 and 70 mg/kg dose (Intraperitoneal) of piperine significantly inhibited (P<0.01) the acetic acid writhing in mice as compared to standard indomethacin (20 mg/kg i.p.). In the tail-flick assay, piperine (30 and 50 mg/kg i.p.) caused a significant increase (P<0.01) in reaction time with a similar effect of standard morphine (5 mg/kg i.p.). Piperine with a dose of 30, 50, and 70 mg/kg i.p. significantly delayed the PTZ and PIC induced seizures in mice. Overall, it was indicated by the author that piperine has good analgesic and anticonvulsant effects possibly mediated *via* opioid and GABAergic pathways, respectively [25].

In another study, Kemao *et al.* (2017) reported that piperine with a dose of 40 mg/kg for continuous 45 days showed the potential 1 to decrease the status epilepticus and prevent memory impairment following pilocarpine-induced epilepsy in rats. The level of caspase-3 and expression level of B-cell lymphoma 2 (Bcl-2) and Bcl-2-associated X protein (Bax) were also suppressed with piperine treatment. Piperine also has the potential to decrease inflammation and free radicals generated due to pilocarpine-induced epilepsy [26].

Anti-Tussive and Bronchodilator Activity

Since the beginning of human civilization, the *Black pepper* is being used for the treatment of respiratory tract infections due to its anti-tussive activity [27]. In an experiment, it was proved that the water extract of *Piper nigrum* (50 mg/kg) containing pectin polysaccharide and piperine has significant anti-tussive activity as compared to codeine phosphate (10 mg/kg). Here it was also reported that pectin polysaccharide has high anti-tussive activity than piperine but if they are used in combination, then piperine provides a synergistic effect to polysaccharides and it shows the most potent anti-tussive activity [28].

In another experiment, Piperine 4.5 and 2.25 mg/kg was orally administered 5 times a week for 8 weeks in asthma induced mice (induced by ovalbumin sensitization and inhalation) and results revealed that piperine has the potential to treat asthma *via* reduction of interleukins-4 and 5, eosinophil infiltration and reduction of thymus and activation regulated chemokine, eotaxin-2 in lung tissue as well as histamine and ovalbumin specific immunoglobulin E production in serum [29].

Anticancer and Antitumor Activity

Ethanolic extract of *Piper nigrum* (50%, 705, and 100%) was evaluated for cytotoxic efficacy against colorectal carcinoma cell lines (HCT-116, HCT-15 and HT-29) based on percentage inhibition of cells using the sulforhodamine-B assay. The results revealed a dose-dependent response curve with maximum cellular inhibition at total phenolic content of 6 and 3 µg/ml with 50% ethanolic extract. However, inhibition of cellular growth decreased with a decrease in total phenolic content, *i.e.* 50% inhibition of cell lines (HCT-15) was seen with phenolic content of 3.2, 2.9, and 1.9 µg/ml at 24, 48 and, 72 hrs, respectively [30].

Extract of *Piper nigrum* without piperine also has a potent anti-tumor effect with low toxicity as revealed in a cytotoxicity study using MTT assay and Western blot analysis. The extract showed selective inhibition against breast cancer cells than colorectal, lung cancer, and neuroblastoma cells [31].

Piperine has also been found to treat prostate cancer. In a study, the author reported that piperine inhibits the growth of LNCaP, PC-3, 22RV1, and DU-145, responsible for the proliferation of prostate cancer cells. Piperine also reduced the secretion of phosphorylated STAT-3 and Nuclear factor –κB transcription factor. Ultimately, it was concluded that piperine significantly reduced androgen-dependent and androgen-independent tumor growth in the mice model xenotransplanted with prostate cancer cells [32]. It was also reported that the piperine arrest cell cycle at G0/G1 down-regulated cyclin D1 and Cyclin A and ultimately inhibited the growth of LNCaP and PC-3 [33]. Furthermore, piperine also improved the antitumor efficacy of docetaxel remarkably in a xenograft model of human castration-resistant prostate cancer [34].

In-vitro cytotoxic activity of Piperine was also evaluated using HeLa Cell lines by MTT assay and 50% inhibition was reported at 61.94 ± 0.054 µg/ml. Piperine was also subjected to molecular docking studies for inhibition of EGFR tyrosine kinase enzyme (an enzyme responsible for cancer cells production); the results revealed -7.6 KJ/mol binding and 7.06 KJ/mol docking energy with 2 hydrogen bonds [35]. The above results strongly suggest that piperine from *Piper nigrum* has the potential to fight against cancerous cells.

Neuroprotective and Antidepressant Activity

Depression is a life-threatening form of mental illness which increases the severity of Alzheimer's disease. Alzheimer's disease is a neurodegenerative disorder of CNS characterized by progressive cognitive dysfunction, *i.e.* change in emotional behavior, enhanced fear, and anxiety [36, 37]. In Alzheimer's disease, excessive deposition of the neurotoxic β-amyloid peptide in the brain causes neuropathological lesions in the brain. Deposition of the β-amyloid peptide is also associated with oxidative stress, *i.e.* elevated level of protein oxidation, lipid peroxidation products and oxidative damage to mitochondria due to the ability of the Aβ peptide to act as a pro-oxidant [38, 39]. So, a study was conducted to evaluate the anxiolytic, antidepressant-like effect of methanolic extract of *Piper nigrum via* elevated plus maze test and forced swimming tests in β-amyloid (1–42) rat model of Alzheimer's disease. Also, the antioxidant activity was analyzed using superoxide dismutase, glutathione peroxidase and catalase specific activities. Results revealed that the methanolic extract of *Black pepper* led to significant depress β-amyloid (1–42) induced anxiolytic depression by controlling free radical generation [40].

Further, it was also reported that piperine, the chief constituent of *Piper nigrum,* has antidepressant-like effect due to its potential to enhance 5-Hydroxytryptamine level (Serotonergic system) in both the hippocampus and frontal cortex of mice [41].

Hepatoprotective Activity and Digestion

Human beings are continuously exposed to different chemicals such as food, industrial chemicals, pesticides, *etc.* which causes injury to biomembranes, cells, and tissues of the liver *via* oxidative stress. Since the liver is a key organ maintaining homeostasis in the body so, it is necessary to protect the liver from the free radicals, and oxidative stress generated due to chemicals. Several studies have been performed to evaluate the hepatoprotective effect of *black pepper* or piperine.

The potential hepatoprotective effect of the ethanolic extract of *Piper nigrum* was shown in a study on ethanol carbon tetrachloride-induced hepatotoxicity. The levels of hepatic biomarkers (Triglycerides (TG), aminotransferases (AST, ALT), alkaline phosphatase (ALP), Bilirubin) decreased with the treatment of extract whereas Superoxide dismutase (SOD), Catalase (CAT), Glutathione reductase (GSH) and lipid peroxidation (TBARS)) levels were increased [42].

Piperine showed a significant hepatoprotective effect when it was evaluated against silymarin in acetaminophen-induced hepatotoxicity in mice. Piperine significantly decreased the levels of hepatic marker enzymes, *i.e.,* [aspartate transaminase (AST), alanine transaminase (ALT), and alkaline phosphatase (ALP)] and Tumor necrosis factor-alpha (TNF-α). The level of lipid peroxidation also decreased with the decrease in free radical generation measured *via* superoxide dismutase, catalase, glutathione peroxidase, glutathione reductase, glutathione-s-transferase, and glutathione [43]. Furthermore, it was also revealed that Piperine in combination with silymarin has more potential to fight against hepatotoxicity [44].

The use of *Black pepper* as a spice with a dose of 1.5 mg/meal caused significant increases in parietal secretion, pepsin secretion, and potassium loss [45]. Piperine with 20 mg dose fed to the animals for 8 weeks resulted in increased intestinal lipase activity and also disaccharidases sucrase and maltase were found to stimulate digestion [46].

PHYTOCHEMICAL STUDIES

The phytochemical studies revealed that the fruit of *Piper nigrum* has alkaloids, glycosides, steroids, flavonoids, tannins, saponins, and terpenoids [47, 48]. The leaf extract of *Piper nigrum* has vitamins and minerals such as vitamin A, vitamin C and vitamin E along with iron, magnesium and selenium. Furthermore, it was also illustrated that 1 gram of leaf extract of *Black pepper* has alkaloids (17.27±0.05 mg/g), steroids (6.06±0.00 mg/g), terpenoids (6.12±0.03 mg/g), flavonoids (9.54±0.05 mg/g), tannins (3.23±0.04 mg/g), and saponins (3.68±0.09 mg/g) along with vitamin A (9.80±0.02 mg/100 g), vitamin C (12.42±0.07 mg/100 g), and vitamin E (7.25±0.03 mg/100 g), Iron (7.28±0.025mg/100g), magnesium (97.58±0.03 mg/100 g), and selenium (1.60±0.025 mg/100) [49]. The extract also contains ascorbic acid, Beta carotene, lauric acid, linalyl acetate, myristic acid, palmitic acid and piperine, responsible for antioxidant activity [50]. The chief constituent of *Black pepper* has piperine, a weak basic substance, not responsible for aroma but imparts pungency to *Black pepper*. Isopiperine, chavicine and isochavicine are isomers of piperine that are also present in the *Black pepper* (Fig. 2). Studies also reveal that seeds of *Black pepper* has\ve about 3.5% of essential oil, which contains sabinene, pinene, phellandrene, linalool and limonene [51, 52].

Ghaidaa *et al.* (2016) investigated the methanolic extract of fruits of *Piper nigrum* and reported 55 bioactive phytochemicals *i.e.* Propanedioic acid, dimethyl ester, Bi-cyclo[3.1.1]heptane,6,6-dimethyl2-methylene-,(1S), 3-Carene, Cyclo hexene, 1-methyl-5-(1-methylethenyl)-,(R), 1,6-Octadien-3-ol,3,7-dimethyl, 2-Methyl-1-ethylpyrrolidine, 2-Isopropenyl-5-methylhex-4-enal, L-α-Terpineol, (R)- lavandulyl acetate, Pyrrolizin-1,7- dione-6-carboxylic acid, methyl(ester), 7-epi-cis-sesquisabinene hydrate, Phenol, 2-methoxy-4-(1-propenyl)-,(Z), Eugenol, Alfa. Copaene, Naphthalene, 1,2,3,5,6,7,8, 8a-octahydro-1,8a-dimethyl-7-(1-methyl), Epiglobulol, Caryophyllene, 1,4,7-Cycloundecatriene, 1,5,9,9 -

tetramethyl-,Z, Z,Z, α-ylangene, ß-copaene, Cedran-diol,8S,13, Isocalamendiol, Cinnamic acid, 4-hydroxy-3-methoxy-,{5-hydroxy-2-hydroxymethyl, (---Spathulenol, 1-Heptatri acotanol, Desacetylanquidine, 5- Isopropyl-2,8-dimeth-l-9-oxatricyclo[4.4.0.0. (2,8)]decan-7-one, Estra-1,3,5(10)-trien-17ß-ol, Trans-1,2- Diaminocyclohexane-N,N,N′,N′-tetraacetic acid, Phytol, Piperidine,1-(--oxo-3-phenyl-2-propenyl)-, Eicosanoic acid, 2-(acetyloxy0-1-[(acetyloxy)methyl]ethyl ester, 2,5,5,8a-Tetramethyl-6,7 ,8,8a-tetr ahydro-5--chromen-8-ol, Z-5-methyl-6-heneicosen-11-one, 2H-1,2-Benzoxazine-3-carbonitri le,2-cyclohexyloctahydro-4a,8a-d, Indoxazin-4-one,4,5,6,7- tetrahydro-3-undecyl, 9,10- Secocholesta-5,7,10(19)-triene-3,24,25-triol,(3ß,5Z,7E), 3-Ox--10(14)- epox yguai -11(13)-en6,12-olide, 7-[2-(Ethoxycarbonyl)-3α-5ß-dimethoxyc yclo pentyl -1] -heptanoic acid, 2H-Benzo[f]oxireno[2,--E]benzofura Piperine, n-8,(9H)-one,9 -[[(1,3-b enz odio, Nalorphine, 2-Cyclohexen-3-ol-1-one, 2-[1-iminotetradecyl] Fenretinide, 11-Dehy drocorticosterone, 5H-Cyclopropa [3, 4]benz[1,2-e]azulen-5-one,1,1a, 1b,4,4a,7a,7b, 17a-Ethyl-3ßmethoxy-17a-aza-D-homoandrost-5-ene-17-one, Buf a-20,22-dienolide,14,15-epoxy-3 ,11-dihy droxy-,(3ß,5ß,11α,15, 9- Desoxo-9-x-acetoxy- 3,8,12-tri-O-ac etyling ol, Retinal, 9-cis-, 6-ß-Naltrexol, Piperine, Ursodeoxycholic acid, 5α-Cholan24-oic acid, 12α-hydroxy-3,7-dioxo-, methyl ester and Stigmasterol (Table **1**) [53].

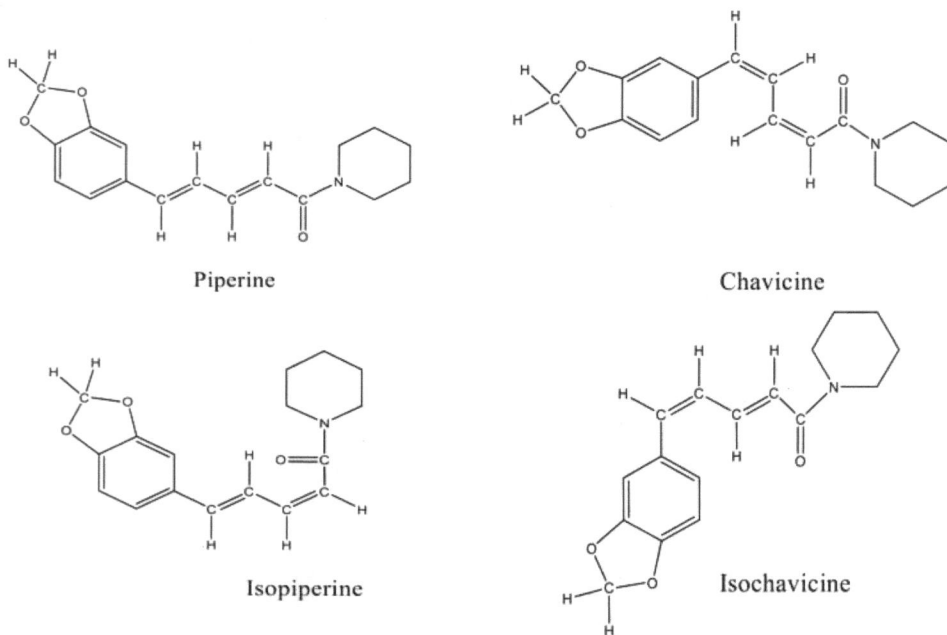

Piperine

Chavicine

Isopiperine

Isochavicine

Fig. (2). Isomers of Piperine.

The aroma of *Black pepper* is due to the presence of piperonal, α-terpineol, Nerol, Nerolidol, Dihydrocarveol and 2-methyl naphthalene. Some more chemicals have also been isolated such as Formylpiperidine, 4-Terpeneol, Aphellandrene epoxide, Carvacrol, 2-Methyl naphthalene, Piperonal, Dimethoxy phenol, Caryophyllene, 2,4-di-tbutylphenol, β–bisabolene, δ–Cadinene, Elemol, Nerolidol, c-murolene, α-Eudesmol, Ethyl linoleate [54, 55].

Table 1. Phytochemicals with Chemical structure.

S. No.	Phytochemical	Chemical Structure
1.	Vitamin A (Beta carotene)	
2.	Vitamin C (Ascorbic acid)	
3.	Vitamin E	
4.	Lauric acid	
5.	Linalyl acetate	
6.	Myristic acid	
7.	Palmitic acid	

(Table 1) cont.....

S. No.	Phytochemical	Chemical Structure
8.	Sabinene	
9.	Pinene	
10.	Phellandrene	
11.	Linalool	
12.	Limonene	
13.	[R]-lavandulyl acetate	
14.	Pyrrolizin-1,7- dione-6-carboxylic acid, methyl ester	
15.	7-epi-cis-sesquisabinene hydrate	
16.	Phenol, 2-methoxy-4-[1-propenyl]-,[Z],	
17.	Eugenol	
18.	Alfa.Copaene	
19.	Naphthalene,1,2,3,5,6,7,8,8a-octahydro-1,8a-dimethyl-7-[1-methyl]	

(Table 1) cont.....

S. No.	Phytochemical	Chemical Structure
20.	Epiglobulol	
21.	Caryophyllene	
22.	1,4,7-Cycloundecatriene, 1,5,9,9-tetramethyl-,Z,Z,Z,	
23.	α- ylangene	
24.	ß-copaene	
25.	Cedran-diol,8S,13-	
26.	Isocalamendiol	
27.	Cinnamic acid 4-hydroxy -3-methoxy-, {5-hydroxy-2-hydroxymethyl,	
28.	[-]-Spathulenol	

(*Table 1*) cont.....

S. No.	Phytochemical	Chemical Structure
29.	1-Heptatriacotanol	
30.	Desacetylanquidine	
31.	5-Isopropyl-2,8-dimethyl-9-oxatricyclo[4.4.0.0 [2, 8].]decan-7-one	
32.	Estra-1,3,5 [10]-trien-17ß-ol	
33.	Trans-1,2- Diaminocyclohexane-N,N,N′,N′-tetraacetic acid	
34.	Phytol	
35.	Piperidine,1-[1-oxo-3-phenyl-2-propenyl]-,	
36.	Eicosanoic acid, 2- [acetyloxy0-1-[[acetyloxy]methyl]ethyl ester	

(Table 1) cont.....

S. No.	Phytochemical	Chemical Structure
37.	2,5,5,8a-Tetramethyl-6,7,8,8a-tetrahydro-5H-chromen-8-ol	
38.	Z-5-methyl-6- heneicosen-11-one	
39.	2H-1,2-Benzoxazine-3-carbonitrile,2- cyclohexyloctahydro-4a,8a-d	
40.	Indoxazin-4-one, 4,5,6,7- tetrahydro-3-undecyl-	
41.	9,10-Secocholesta-5,7,10 [19]-triene-3,24,25-triol,[3ß,5Z,7E]-	
42.	3-Oxo-10 [14]-epoxyguai-11 [13]-en 6,12-olide	
43.	7-[2-[Ethoxycarbonyl]-3α,5ß-dimethoxycyclopentyl -1]-heptanoic acid	

(Table 1) cont.....

S. No.	Phytochemical	Chemical Structure
44.	2H-Benzo[f]oxireno[2,3- E]benzofuran-8,[9H]-one,9-[[[-,3-benzodio	
45.	Nalorphine	
46.	2-Cyclohexen -3-ol-1-one, 2-[1-iminotetradecyl]-,	
47.	Fenretinide	
48.	11-Dehydrocorticosterone	
49.	5H-Cyclopropa [3, 4]benz[1,2-e]azulen-5-one,1,1a,1b,4,4a,7a,7b	
50.	17a-Ethyl-3ßmethoxy-17a-aza-D-homoandrost-5-ene-17-one	

(Table 1) cont.....

S. No.	Phytochemical	Chemical Structure
51.	Bufa-20,22-dienolide m,14,15-epoxy-3,11-dihydr-xy-,[3ß,5ß,11α,15	
52.	9-Desoxo-9-x-acetoxy-3,8,12-tri-O-acetylingol	
53.	Bicyclo[3.1.1]heptane,6,6-dimethyl2-methylene-,[1S]	
54.	Propanedioic acid, dimethyl ester	
55.	Cyclohexene, 1-methyl-5-[1-methylethenyl]-,[R]	
56.	1,6-Octadien-3-ol, 3,7-dimethyl	
57.	L-α-Terpineol	
58.	3-Carene	
59.	Retinal, 9-cis-,	
60.	6-ß-Naltrexol	

(Table 1) cont.....

S. No.	Phytochemical	Chemical Structure
61.	Stigmasterol	
62.	5α-Cholan-24-oic acid, 12α-hydroxy-3,7-dioxo-,methyl ester	
63.	2- Methyl-1-ethylpyrrolidine	
64.	2-Isopropenyl-5-methylhex-4-enal	

HERBAL FORMULATIONS (TABLE 2)

Black pepper is used as a spice and available in the market as a whole as well as a powdered, dried fruit. Different herbal formulations are available in the market employing a basic ayurvedic healing concept. Herbal formulation in the name of "Trikatu" is also available in the market, and is marketed by different companies. Trikatu is a mixture of equal parts of each fruit of *Black pepper* (*Piper nigrum*), long pepper (*Piper longum*) and rhizomes of Ginger (*Zingiber officinale*). It is used to maintain normal gastric function and normal circulation [56].

An ayurvedic formulation "Hingwashtak Churna" is also available in the market having eight ingredients each in equal part, *i.e.* *Piper nigrum*, Piper longum, *Zingiber officinale, Nigella sativa, Cuminum cyminum, Trachyspermum ammi, Ferula foetida* and Rock salt. The formulation is mainly used for flatulence, indigestion, constipation and other disorders related to impaired metabolism of the digestive tract [57].

A polyherbal formulation, Avipattikar churna, used for the treatment of peptic ulcer has 14 different ingredients, *i.e.* Shunthi *(Zingiber officinale)*, Maricha *(Piper nigrum)*, Pippali *(Piper longum)*, Haritaki *(Terminalia chebula)*, Vibhitaka *(Terminalia bellerica)*, Aamalaki *(Emblica officinalis)*, Musta *(Cyperus rotundus)*, salt *(Vida Lavana)*, Vidanga *(Embelia ribes)*, Ela *(Amomum subulatum)*, Patra *(Cinnamomum tamala)*, Lavanga *(Syzgium aromaticum)*, Trivrit *(Operculina terpethum)* and Sharkara (Sugar candy). All the components are present in 1 part except Lavanga, Trivrit and Sugar candy, which are present in 11, 44 and 66 parts, respectively [58].

Talisadya churna, an ancient ayurvedic formulation used for vomiting, flatulence with a gurgling sound, cough, asthma, fever, anorexia, indigestion, diarrhea, cachexia, splenic disease, malabsorption syndrome, and anemia, constitutes Talisa (*Abies webbiana*), Maricha (*Piper nigrum*), Shunti (*Zingiber officinale*), Pippali (*Piper logum*), Vamshalochana (*Bambusa bambos*), Ela (*Elettaria cardamomum*), Twak (*Cinnamomum zelyanicum*), Sharkara (Cane sugar) [59].

A polyherbal formulation is used as a carminative, an antispasmodic, is helpful in all painful conditions like sciatica and stiffness in back and also restores normal digestive functions known as Ajomdadi churna constituted *Trachyspermum ammi, Piper nigrum, Piper longum, Plumbago zeylanica, Terminalia chebula, Cedrus deodara, P. longum* (stems), salt (Saindava lavana), *Embelia ribes, Zingiber officinale, Argyreia nervosa,* and *Anethum graveolens* [60].

Lasunadivati, an ayurvedic formulation, consists of *Alium sativum, Cuminumcyminum*, Rock salt, Gandhak, *Zingiber officinalis, Piper longum, Piper nigrum*, Asafetida and lemon juice. It is used for the treatment of dyspepsia, digestion and diarrhea. It is also helpful for lowering cholesterol and obesity [61].

Marichyadivati, an ayurvedic formulation, contains 2 herbs Piper longum and *Piper nigrum* along with yavaksara, dadima and guda. The formulation is used for the treatment of cough and asthma [62].

Several Unani formulations in the name of Hab-e-Azarakhi, Jawarish-e-Bisbasa and Habb-e- Khardel are also available in the market. Some formulations having piperine, the chief constituent of *Black pepper,* are also available such as "Vista nutrition" and "Zenith nutrition" having curcumin along with piperine. Curcumin has anti-oxidant and anti-inflammatory effects. Curcumin with Piperine helps in maintaining a healthy liver and protecting the brain cells [63].

Majeed *et al.* (1999) reported that piperine, the chief constituent of *Black pepper,* is widely used in various herbal cough syrups due to its potent anti-tussive and bronchodilator properties. It is used in anti-inflammatory, anti-malarial, and anti-leukemia treatment. Recently, medical studies have shown that it is helpful in increasing the absorption of certain vitamins, selenium, β-carotene, also increasing the body's natural thermogenic activity [27].

Table 2. Herbal formulations of Black Pepper.

S. No.	Herbal Formulation	Ingredients along with Black Pepper	Uses
1.	Trikatu	*Black pepper* [*Piper nigrum*], long pepper [*Piper longum*], Ginger [*Zingiber officinale*].	It is used to maintain normal gastric function and normal circulation.
2.	Hingwashtak Churna	*Piper nigrum, Piper longum, Zingiber officinale, Nigella sativa, Cuminum cyminum, Trachyspermum ammi, Ferula foetida,* Rock salt	The formulation is mainly used for flatulence, indigestion, constipation and other disorders related to impaired metabolism of the digestive tract.
3.	Avipattikar churna	*Zingiber officinale, Piper nigrum, Piper longum,* Terminalia chebula, Vibhitaka [*Terminalia bellerica*], Aamalaki [*Emblica officinalis*], Musta [*Cyperus rotundus*], salt [*Vida Lavana*], Vidanga [*Embelia ribes*], Ela [*Amomum subulatum*], Patra [*Cinnamomum tamala*], Lavanga [*Syzgium aromaticum*], Trivrit [*Operculina terpethum*] and Sharkara [*Sugar candy*].	Used for the treatment of peptic ulcer.
4.	Talisadya churna	Talisa [Abies webbiana], Maricha [*Piper nigrum*], Shunti [*Zingiber officinale*], Pippali [*Piper logum*], Vamshalochana [*Bambusa bambos*], Ela [*Elettaria cardamomum*], Twak [*Cinnamomum zelyanicum*], Sharkara [Cane sugar].	Used for vomiting, flatulence with a gurgling sound, cough, asthma, fever, anorexia, indigestion, diarrhea, cachexia, splenic disease, malabsorption syndrome, anaemia.
5.	Ajomdadi churna	*Trachyspermum ammi, Piper nigrum, Piper longum, Plumbago zeylanica, Terminalia chebula, Cedrus deodara, P. longum* [stems], salt [Saindava lavana], *Embelia ribes, Zingiber officinale, Argyreia nervosa,* and *Anethum graveolens*	Used as a carminative, an antispasmodic, being helpful in all painful conditions like sciatica and stiffness in back, and also restores normal digestive functions.
6.	Lasunadi vati	Alium sativum, Cuminum cyminum, Rock salt, Gandhak, *Zingiber officinalis, Piper longum, Piper nigrum,* Asafoetida and lemon juice.	It is used for the treatment of dyspepsia, digestion and diarrhea. It also lowers cholestrol and obesity.
7.	Marichyadi vati	Piper longum and *Piper nigrum* along with yavaksara, dadima and guda.	The formulation is used for the treatment of cough and asthma.

TRADITIONAL AND ETHNOMEDICINAL USES

Black pepper is one of the world's oldest and most venerable spices and has played a key role throughout history for thousands of years. Historically used as both a spice and medicine, *Black pepper* has many traditional uses as a digestive aid, for the treatment of gastrointestinal disorders and as a preserving agent. In the literature, there are many reviews on traditional and ethnomedicinal uses of *Black pepper*. *Black pepper* is traditionally used as an antioxidant, antimicrobial, anti-inflammatory, gastro-protective and antidepressant, antiseptic, antispasmodic, aromatic, analgesic, anti-toxicant, aphrodisiac, antipyretic agent, for rheumatism, diabetes, muscular ache, as diuretic, flavor, spirit, in dyspepsia, to increase salivary secretion and promote digestion, as CNS stimulant, for indigestion and flatulence, throat ache, cold, as germicidal, blood purifier, antibacterial, religious value, in cancer, pungency, kitchen curry, cough, as carminative, insecticide, *etc.* [1, 64, 65].

In Ayurveda, *Black pepper* has been mixed with castor oil, cow's urine or ghee for treating stomach ailments such as dyspepsia, flatulence, constipation and diarrhea. The tablets of *Black pepper* are used for cholera and syphilis, and also chewed to reduce throat inflammation. Externally, it has been applied as a paste to boils, to treat hair loss and for some skin diseases. Oil of pepper is reputed to alleviate itching with a mixture of sesame oil. The powdered *Black pepper* has been recommended for application to areas affected by paralysis. A mixture of *Black pepper* and honey is regarded as a remedy for night blindness. *Black pepper* is also given by inhalation to comatose patients. It is also believed to be useful against hepatitis, urinary and reproductive disorders [66].

CONCLUSION

After compiling different research articles on *Black pepper,* it was revealed that *Black pepper* has significant potential to fight against various ailments and diseases. It possesses antioxidant, antimicrobial, antidiarrheal, analgesic, anti-inflammatory, anticonvulsant, anti-tussive, bronchodilator, anticancer, antidepressant, hepatoprotective, digestive and antipyretic activities. Piperine is the major bioactive constituent of *Black pepper*. Piperine has also been found to increase the absorption of many drugs and has shown bioavailability, enhancing the activity of many drugs and nutrients. This important property of piperine may be very helpful to enhance the therapeutic efficacy of many therapeutically important drugs. Piperine possesses antihypertensive and antiplatelets, antioxidant, antitumor, anti-asthmatic, antipyretic, analgesic, anti-inflammatory, anti-diarrheal, antispasmodic, anxiolytic, antidepressant, hepato-protective, immuno-modulatory, antibacterial, antifungal, anti-thyroid, antiapoptotic, anti-metastatic, antimutagenic, anti-spermatogenic, anti-colon toxin, insecticidal and larvicidal activities.

The phytochemical studies of *Black pepper* have revealed that it has more than 500 phytochemicals that chiefly belong to alkaloids, glycosides, steroids, flavonoids, tannins, saponins and terpenoids. The leaf extract of *Piper nigrum* has vitamins and minerals such as vitamin A, vitamin C and vitamin E along with iron, magnesium and selenium.

Several herbal formulations are available in the market involving *Black pepper* as an ingredient such as trikatu, hingwashtak churna, avipattikar churna, talisadya churna, ajomdadi churna, *etc.* All information deduced on medicinal and nutritional value, and phytochemical constituents of *Black pepper* has been included in this chapter, which will find its utility in the academic field, scientific research and real-world industrial applications.

CONSENT FOR PUBLICATION

Not applicable.

CONFLICT OF INTEREST

The authors confirm that there is no conflict of interest.

ACKNOWLEDGEMENTS

None Declared.

REFERENCES

[1]   Joshi DR, Shrestha AC, Adhikari N. A review on diversified use of the king of spices: *Piper nigrum*. Int J Pharm Sci Res 2018; 9(10): 4089-101.

[2]   Ahmad N, Fazal H, Abbasi BH, Farooq S, Ali M, Khan MA. Biological role of *Piper nigrum* L. [*Black pepper*]: A review. Asian Pac J Trop Biomed 2012; S1945-53.
         [http://dx.doi.org/10.1016/S2221-1691(12)60524-3]

[3]   Acharya SG, Momin AH, Gajjar AV. Review of piperine as a bioenhancer. Am J Pharm Tech Res 2012; 2: 32-44.

[4]   Taqvi SI, Shah AJ, Gilani AH. Blood pressure lowering and vasomodulator effects of piperine. J Cardiovasc Pharmacol 2008; 52(5): 452-8.
         [http://dx.doi.org/10.1097/FJC.0b013e31818d07c0] [PMID: 19033825]

[5]   Manoharan S, Balakrishnan S, Menon VP, Alias LM, Reena AR. Chemopreventive efficacy of curcumin and piperine during 7,12-dimethylbenz[a]anthracene-induced hamster buccal pouch carcinogenesis. Singapore Med J 2009; 50(2): 139-46.
         [PMID: 19296028]

[6]   Parganiha R, Verma S, Chandrakar S, Pal S, Sawarkar HA, Kashyap P. *In-vitro* anti- asthmatic activity of fruit extract of *Piper nigrum*. Inter J Herbal Drug Res 2011; 1: 15-8.

[7]   Li S, Wang C, Wang M, Li W, Matsumoto K, Tang Y. Antidepressant like effects of piperine in chronic mild stress treated mice and its possible mechanisms. Life Sci 2007; 80(15): 1373-81.
         [http://dx.doi.org/10.1016/j.lfs.2006.12.027] [PMID: 17289085]

[8]   Matsuda H, Ninomiya K, Morikawa T, Yasuda D, Yamaguchi I, Yoshikawa M. Protective effects of amide constituents from the fruit of Piper chaba on D-galactosamine/TNF-alpha-induced cell death in mouse hepatocytes. Bioorg Med Chem Lett 2008; 18(6): 2038-42.

[http://dx.doi.org/10.1016/j.bmcl.2008.01.101] [PMID: 18289853]

[9] Damanhouri ZA, Ahmad A. A Review on Therapeutic Potential of *Piper nigrum* L. [*Black pepper*]: The King of Spices. Med Aromat Plants 2014; 3: 3.
[http://dx.doi.org/10.4172/2167-0412.1000161]

[10] Shaheen N, Imam S, Sultan RA, Abidi S, Azhar I, Mahmood ZA. Pharmacognostic Evaluation and Instrumental Analysis [sem] for the standardization of *Piper nigrum* l., [*Black pepper*] fruit. Pak J Bot 2019; 51(5): 1859-63.
[http://dx.doi.org/10.30848/PJB2019-5(32)]

[11] Gülçin I. The antioxidant and radical scavenging activities of *black pepper* (*Piper nigrum*) seeds. Int J Food Sci Nutr 2005; 56(7): 491-9.
[http://dx.doi.org/10.1080/09637480500450248] [PMID: 16503560]

[12] Nahak G, Sahu RK. Phytochemical Evaluation and Antioxidant activity of *Piper cubeba* and *Piper nigrum*. J Appl Pharm Sci 2011; 01(08): 153-7.

[13] Sapam R, Kalita PP, Sarma MP, Talukdar N, Das H. Screening of phytochemicals and determination of total phenolic content, anti-oxidant, and antimicrobial activity of methanolic extract of *Piper nigrum* leaves. Indo Am J Pharm Res 2018; 8(2): 1354-60.

[14] Mahady GB, Huang Y, Doyle BJ. Natural products as antibacterial agents. Studies in natural products chemistry. Elsevier BV. 2008.
[http://dx.doi.org/10.1016/S1572-5995(08)80011-7]

[15] Abdallah EM, Abdalla WE. *Black pepper* fruit [*Piper nigrum* L.] as antibacterial agent: A mini-review. J Bacteriol Mycol Open Access 2018; 6(2): 141-5.
[http://dx.doi.org/10.15406/jbmoa.2018.06.00192]

[16] Zou L, Hu YY, Chen WX. Antibacterial mechanism and activities of black pepper chloroform extract. J Food Sci Technol 2015; 52(12): 8196-203.
[http://dx.doi.org/10.1007/s13197-015-1914-0] [PMID: 26604394]

[17] Kaho ZM, Kadum AR, Hadi AA. Evalution of antibacterial activity of *Piper nigrum* extract against *Streptococcus mutans* and *Escherichia coli*. J Pharm Sci & Res 2019; 11(2): 367-70.

[18] Shamkuwar PB, Shahi SR, Jadhav ST. Evaluation of antidiarrhoeal effect of *Black pepper*. Asian J Plant Sci 2012; 2(1): 48-53.

[19] Shamkuwar PB. Mechanisms of Antidiarrhoeal Effect of *Piper nigrum*. Int J Pharm Tech Res 2013; 5(3): 1138-41.

[20] Mehmood MH, Gilani AH. Pharmacological basis for the medicinal use of *black pepper* and piperine in gastrointestinal disorders. J Med Food 2010; 13(5): 1086-96.
[http://dx.doi.org/10.1089/jmf.2010.1065] [PMID: 20828313]

[21] Tasleem F, Azhar I, Ali S N, Perveen S, Mahmood Z A. Analgesic and anti-inflammatory activities of *Piper nigrum* L. Asian Pac J Trop Med 2014; 61-8. 7S1:S4

[22] Wanga B, Zhanga Y, Huanga J, Donga L, Lic T, Fu X. Anti-inflammatory activity and chemical composition of dichloromethane extract from *Piper nigrum* and P.longum on permanent focal cerebral ischemia injury in rats. Rev Bras Farmacogn 2017; 27: 369-74.
[http://dx.doi.org/10.1016/j.bjp.2017.02.003]

[23] Bang JS, Oh DH, Choi HM, *et al.* Anti-inflammatory and antiarthritic effects of piperine in human interleukin 1β-stimulated fibroblast-like synoviocytes and in rat arthritis models. Arthritis Res Ther 2009; 11(2): R49.
[http://dx.doi.org/10.1186/ar2662] [PMID: 19327174]

[24] Sabina EP, Nasreen A, Vedi M, Rasool MK. Analgesic, antipyretic and ulcerogenic effects of piperine: an active ingredient of pepper. J Pharm Sci & Res 2013; 5(10): 203-6.

[25] Bukhari IA, Pivac N, Alhumayyd MS, Mahesar AL, Gilani AH. The analgesic and anticonvulsant

effects of piperine in mice. J Physiol Pharmacol 2013; 64(6): 789-94.
[PMID: 24388894]

[26]   Mao K, Lei D, Zhang H, You C. Anticonvulsant effect of piperine ameliorates memory impairment, inflammation and oxidative stress in a rat model of pilocarpine-induced epilepsy. Exp Ther Med 2017; 13(2): 695-700.
[http://dx.doi.org/10.3892/etm.2016.4001] [PMID: 28352353]

[27]   Majeed M, Badmeev V, Rajendran R. Use of piperine as a bioavailability enhancer. United State Patent 1999; ([5]): 382-972.

[28]   Khawas S, Nosáľová G, Majee SK, *et al. In vivo* cough suppressive activity of pectic polysaccharide with arabinogalactan type II side chains of *Piper nigrum* fruits and its synergistic effect with piperine. Int J Biol Macromol 2017; 99: 335-42.
[http://dx.doi.org/10.1016/j.ijbiomac.2017.02.093] [PMID: 28254575]

[29]   Kim SH, Lee YC. Piperine inhibits eosinophil infiltration and airway hyperresponsiveness by suppressing T cell activity and Th2 cytokine production in the ovalbumin-induced asthma model. J Pharm Pharmacol 2009; 61(3): 353-9.
[http://dx.doi.org/10.1211/jpp.61.03.0010] [PMID: 19222908]

[30]   Prashant A, Rangaswamy C, Yadav AK, Reddy V, Sowmya MN, Madhunapantula S. *In vitro* anticancer activity of ethanolic extracts of *Piper nigrum* against colorectal carcinoma cell lines. Int J Appl Basic Med Res 2017; 7(1): 67-72.
[http://dx.doi.org/10.4103/2229-516X.198531] [PMID: 28251112]

[31]   Sriwiriyajan S, Tedasen A, Lailerd N, *et al.* Anticancer and cancer prevention effects of piperine-free *Piper nigrum* extract on n-nitrosomethylurea-induced mammary tumorigenesis in rats. Cancer Prev Res (Phila) 2016; 9(1): 74-82.
[http://dx.doi.org/10.1158/1940-6207.CAPR-15-0127] [PMID: 26511488]

[32]   Samykutty A, Shetty AV, Dakshinamoorthy G, *et al.* Piperine, a bioactive component of pepper spice exerts therapeutic effects on androgen dependent and androgen independent prostate cancer cells. PLoS One 2013; 8(6): e65889.
[http://dx.doi.org/10.1371/journal.pone.0065889] [PMID: 23824300]

[33]   Ouyang DY, Zeng LH, Pan H, *et al.* Piperine inhibits the proliferation of human prostate cancer cells *via* induction of cell cycle arrest and autophagy. Food Chem Toxicol 2013; 60: 424-30.
[http://dx.doi.org/10.1016/j.fct.2013.08.007] [PMID: 23939040]

[34]   Makhov P, Golovine K, Canter D, *et al.* Co-administration of piperine and docetaxel results in improved anti-tumor efficacy *via* inhibition of CYP3A4 activity. Prostate 2012; 72(6): 661-7.
[http://dx.doi.org/10.1002/pros.21469] [PMID: 21796656]

[35]   Paarakh PM, Sreeram DC, D SS, Ganapathy SPS. *In vitro* cytotoxic and in silico activity of piperine isolated from *Piper nigrum* fruits Linn. In Silico Pharmacol 2015; 3(1): 9.
[http://dx.doi.org/10.1186/s40203-015-0013-2] [PMID: 26820894]

[36]   Wuwongse S, Chang RC-C, Law ACK. The putative neurodegenerative links between depression and Alzheimer's disease. Prog Neurobiol 2010; 91(4): 362-75.
[http://dx.doi.org/10.1016/j.pneurobio.2010.04.005] [PMID: 20441786]

[37]   Seignourel PJ, Kunik ME, Snow L, Wilson N, Stanley M. Anxiety in dementia: a critical review. Clin Psychol Rev 2008; 28(7): 1071-82.
[http://dx.doi.org/10.1016/j.cpr.2008.02.008] [PMID: 18555569]

[38]   Suh Y-H, Checler F. Amyloid precursor protein, presenilins, and α-synuclein: molecular pathogenesis and pharmacological applications in Alzheimer's disease. Pharmacol Rev 2002; 54(3): 469-525.
[http://dx.doi.org/10.1124/pr.54.3.469] [PMID: 12223532]

[39]   Martorell P, Bataller E, Llopis S, *et al.* A cocoa peptide protects *Caenorhabditis elegans* from oxidative stress and β-amyloid peptide toxicity. PLoS One 2013; 8(5): e63283.

[http://dx.doi.org/10.1371/journal.pone.0063283] [PMID: 23675471]

[40]   Hritcu L, Noumedem JA, Cioanca O, Hancianu M, Postu P, Mihasan M. Anxiolytic and antidepressant profile of the methanolic extract of *Piper nigrum* fruits in beta-amyloid (1-42) rat model of Alzheimer's disease. Behav Brain Funct 2015; 11: 13.
[http://dx.doi.org/10.1186/s12993-015-0059-7] [PMID: 25880991]

[41]   Mao QQ, Xian YF, Ip SP, Che CT. Involvement of serotonergic system in the antidepressant-like effect of piperine. Prog Neuropsychopharmacol Biol Psychiatry 2011; 35(4): 1144-7.
[http://dx.doi.org/10.1016/j.pnpbp.2011.03.017] [PMID: 21477634]

[42]   Nirwane AM, Bapat AR. Effect of methanolic extract of *Piper nigrum* fruits in Ethanol-CCl4 induced hepatotoxicity in Wistar rats. Der Pharmacia Lettre 2012; 4(3): 795-802.

[43]   Sabina EP, Deborah A, Souriyan H, Jackline D, Rasool MK. Piperine, an active ingredient of *Black pepper* attenuates acetaminophen-induced hepatotoxicity in mice. Asian Pac J Trop Med 2010; 3(12): 971-6.
[http://dx.doi.org/10.1016/S1995-7645(11)60011-4]

[44]   Shukla R, Surana SJ, Tatiya AU, Das SK. Investigation of hepatoprotective effects of piperine and silymarin on D-galactosamine induced hepatotoxicity in rats. Res J Pharm Biol Chem Sci 2011; 2(3): 975-82.

[45]   Myers BM, Smith JL, Graham DY. Effect of red pepper and *black pepper* on the stomach. Am J Gastroenterol 1987; 82(3): 211-4.
[PMID: 3103424]

[46]   Platel K, Srinivasan K. Influence of dietary spices or their active principles on digestive enzymes of small intestinal mucosa in rats. Int J Food Sci Nutr 1996; 47(1): 55-9.
[http://dx.doi.org/10.3109/09637489609028561] [PMID: 8616674]

[47]   Jyothiprabha V, Venkatachalam P. Preliminary phytochemical screening of different solvent extracts of selected Indian spices. Int J Curr Microbiol Appl Sci 2016; 5(2): 116-22.
[http://dx.doi.org/10.20546/ijcmas.2016.502.013]

[48]   Shetty S, Vijayalaxmi K K. Phytochemical investigation of extract/ solvent fractions of *Piper nigrum* linn. Seeds and piper betle linn. Leaves. Int J Pharma Bio Sci 2012; 3(2): 344-9.

[49]   Onyesife CO, Ogugua VN, Anaduaka EG. Investigation of some important phytochemicals, vitamins and mineral constituents of ethanol leaves extract of *Piper nigrum.* Ann Biol Res 2014; 5(6): 20-5.

[50]   Srinivasan K. Spices as influencers of body metabolism: an overview of three decades of research. Food Res Int 2005; 38: 77-86.
[http://dx.doi.org/10.1016/j.foodres.2004.09.001]

[51]   Ahluwalia VK, Raghav S. Comprihensive experimental chemistry. New Delhi: Arya publishers 1997.

[52]   Vijayan KK, Thampuran RVA. Pharmacology, toxicology and clinical applications of Black pepper. Harwood Academic Publishers 2000.

[53]   Ghaidaa JM, Omran AS, Hussein HM. Antibacterial and Phytochemical Analysis of *Piper nigrum* using Gas Chromatography – Mass Spectrum and Fourier-Transform Infrared Spectroscopy. Int. J Pharmacog. Phytochem Rev 2016; 8(6): 977-96.

[54]   Gupta M, Gupta A, Gupta S. *In-vitro* antimicrobial and phytochemical analysis of dichloromethane extracts of *Piper nigrumBlack pepper.* Orient J Chem 2013; 29(2): 777-82.
[http://dx.doi.org/10.13005/ojc/290259]

[55]   Murthy CT, Bhattacharya S. Cryogenic grinding of *Black pepper.* J Food Eng 2008; 85: 18-28.
[http://dx.doi.org/10.1016/j.jfoodeng.2007.06.020]

[56]   Johri RK, Zutshi U. An Ayurvedic formulation 'Trikatu' and its constituents. J Ethnopharmacol 1992; 37(2): 85-91.
[http://dx.doi.org/10.1016/0378-8741(92)90067-2] [PMID: 1434692]

[57]   Pal RS, Pal Y, Wal P, Wal A. In house & Marketed Preparation of Hingwashtak Churna, A Polyherbal Formulation: Comparative Standardization and Measures. Open Med J 2018; 5: 76-83.
[http://dx.doi.org/10.2174/1874220301805010076]

[58]   Gyawali S, Khan GM, Lamichane S, *et al.* Evaluation of anti-secretory and anti-ulcerogenic activities of avipattikar churna on the peptic ulcers in experimental rats. J Clin Diagn Res 2013; 7(6): 1135-9.
[http://dx.doi.org/10.7860/JCDR/2013/5309.3058] [PMID: 23905120]

[59]   Jain P, Pandey R, Shukla SS. Acute and subacute toxicity studies of polyherbal formulation of talisadya churna in experimental animal model. Mintage J Pharma Med Sci 2015; 1 (Suppl. 1): 7-10.

[60]   Sriwastava NK, Shreedhara CS, Aswatha Ram HN. Standardization of Ajmodadi churna, a polyherbal formulation. Pharmacognosy Res 2010; 2(2): 98-101.
[http://dx.doi.org/10.4103/0974-8490.62957] [PMID: 21808548]

[61]   https://ayurmedinfo.com/2012/06/30/lashunadi-vati-benefits-dosage-ingredients-and-side-effects/

[62]   Khan P I, Bhandari A, Kumar A. Standardization of Ayurvedic Formulation [Marichyadi Vati] Using HPLC and HPTLC Methods. World Academy of Science, Engineering and Technology Int J Pharmacol Pharmaceu Sci 2014; 8(4).

[63]   Chopra B, Dhingra AK, Kapoor RP, Prasad DN. Piperine and its various physicochemical and biological aspects: a review. Open Chem J 2016; 3: 75-96.
[http://dx.doi.org/10.2174/1874842201603010075]

[64]   Balasubramanian S, Roselin P, Singh KK, Zachariah J, Saxena SN. Postharvest processing and benefits of *Black pepper*, coriander, cinnamon, fenugreek, and turmeric spices. Crit Rev Food Sci Nutr 2016; 56(10): 1585-607.
[http://dx.doi.org/10.1080/10408398.2012.759901] [PMID: 25747463]

[65]   Butt MS, Pasha I, Sultan MT, Randhawa MA, Saeed F, Ahmed W. *Black pepper* and health claims: a comprehensive treatise. Crit Rev Food Sci Nutr 2013; 53(9): 875-86.
[http://dx.doi.org/10.1080/10408398.2011.571799] [PMID: 23768180]

[66]   Asavirama P, Upender M. Piperine: A valuable alkaloid from piper species. Int J Pharm Pharm Sci 2014; 6: 34-8.

CHAPTER 7

Coriander: A Herb with Multiple Benefits

Ashish Singhai[1], Vipin Dhote[1] and **Aman Upaganlawar[2],***

[1] *Faculty of Pharmacy, VNS Group of Institutions, Bhopal: 462044, India*

[2] *SNJB's SSDJ College of Pharmacy, Neminagar, Chandwad, Maharashtra 423101, India*

Abstract: *Coriandrum sativum* is an aromatic, glabrous, and annual herb of height 30-90 cm belonging to family Apiaceae. Its volatile oil content (~1%) has linalool (60-70%) as a major component, and also has limonene, borneol, phenolic acid, citronellol, and flavonoids, *etc.* Conventionally, it is used for various purposes, for example. in inflammatory bowel diseases, post-coital anti-fertility activity, anxiety relief, sleeping disorder, and a digestive aid. It is also known for its various pharmacological properties, such as antibacterial, anti-mutagenic, anxiolytic effect, anthelmintic, antioxidant, acute diuretic. Storage of ground coriander should be in an opaque and tightly closed container as it loses aroma and flavor quickly. It synergizes the pharmacological effects with certain oils, including eucalyptus and dill oil. Various clinical studies also highlight the evidence generated by preclinical investigations. This study on *Coriandrum sativum* deals with the compilation of its vast pharmacological applications with pharmacognostic and phytochemical information, as it is gaining importance as a therapeutically effective medicinal agent from various scientific reports.

Keywords: Anthelmintic Activity, Antioxidants, Antibacterial Activity, Anxiolytic Effect, Antimutagenic Activity, *Coriandrum sativum*, Post Coital Antifertility Activity.

INTRODUCTION

The essential oils and extracts of aromatic plants and spices are used in food preservation, pharmaceuticals, alternative medicine, and natural therapies. Currently, it is necessary to investigate those plants scientifically for their biological activities, which have been used in traditional medicine to improve the quality of healthcare. Additionally, the conservation of biodiversity can be supported by studying a classical plant systematically. This aspect of cultivated plants and their diversity at certain levels is still overlooked. So for all future res-

* **Corresponding author Aman Upaganlawar:** SNJB's SSDJ College of Pharmacy, Neminagar, Chandwad, Maharashtra 423101, India; Tel: +917774039184; E-mail: amanrxy@gmail.com

Atta-ur-Rahman, M. Iqbal Choudhary & Sammer Yousuf (Eds.)

earches and developmental studies, it becomes necessary to systematically describe the cultivated species, which are of interest to consumers and growers. And the updates on the usefulness of medicinal and aromatic plant *e.g. Coriandrum sativum* should be based on the scientific studies for the benefit of mankind.

TAXONOMY

The Coriandreae tribe is relatively small: it belongs to subfamily Apioideae. Most of its genera are included in Umbelliferae and originated in the temperate areas of Asia and Europe. This family has 455 genera and 3600-3751 species, the tribe Coriandereae has 8 genera and 21species. The genera are *Bifora, Coriandrum, Fuernrohria, Kosopoljanskia, Lipskya, Schrenkia, Schtschurowskia* and *Sclerotiari.*

The six other genera of the tribe Coriandreae, wild plants from Central Asia, are perennials and have quite different morphology from coriander, according to the comparison with herbarium specimens at the Botanical Institute in St. Petersburg.

Coriandrum sativum (*C. Sativum*) and *C. tordyliu* (CT) are the cultivated plants and the wild species of the genus Coriandrum, respectively. CT is native to northern Lebanon and southeastern Anatolia. The other morphologically similar variety of coriander, *Bifora radians,* has different shapes of fruits and does not contain essential oil, whereas it is rich in fatty oil content *e.g.* 49.5%. *B. radians* (german name- 'Getreideverpester' or 'cereal polluter') is a green plant with a very strong unpleasant smell, considered a weed as it affects the growth of cereals with which it grows.

Coriandrum sativum is an annual herb of the Apiaceae family. For culinary purposes, either the fruits (as a spice) or the leaves (as a herb) of this plant are used, known as 'Coriander'. This herbaceous annual plant is aromatic and glabrous [1]. 'Coriander' name is derived from the French and Latin words 'coriandre' and 'coriandrum' [2], while some naming records from John Chadwick show its origination from the greek word koriadnon (name of the Minos daughter Ariadne), which got its name koriannon or koriandron, later [3]. It has various botanical names and synonyms *e.g. Coriandrum majus* Gouan (1762), *Coriandrum diversifolium* Gilib. (1782), *Coriandrum testiculatum* Lour. (1790), *Coriandrum globosum* Salisb. (1796), *Bifora loureirii* Kostel. (1835), *Coriandrum melphitense* Ten. (1837) and *Selinum coriandrum* (1904*).* Some of the common names are enlisted in Table **1**.

Table 1. Common names of Coriander.

Language	Names
Arab	kuzbara, kuzbura
Armenian	Chamem
Chinese	yuan sui, hu sui
Czech	Koriandr
Danish	koriander
Dutch	koriander
English	coriander, collender, chinese parsley
Ethiopian (Amharic)	Dembilal
French	coriandre, persil arabe
Greek	koriannon, korion
Hindi	dhania, dhanya
Russian	koriandr, koljandra, ki nec, kinza, vonju ee zel'e, klopovnik
German	Koriander, Wanzendill, Schwindelkorn
Sanskrit	dhanayaka, kusthumbari

The cultivated or wild status of the coriander plant was commented by Zohary and Hopf, as it is wildly grown in wide areas of the Near East and Southern Europe. They elucidated that it is not easy to define whether it is wild or not [4].

HISTORIC OCCURRENCE

Archeologically, the 15 desiccated mericarps, found in the Pre-Pottery Neolithic B level of the Nahal Hemel Cave in Israel, were considered the oldest finding. Mericarps of coriander were also recovered from the tomb of Tutankhamun; Zohary and Hopf interpreted that coriander was cultivated by ancient Egyptians because this plant does not grow wildly there [4]. Coriander is mentioned in the Bible in Exodus 16:31, and there is also reference to its cultivation in Greece, since at least the second millennium BC [5]. Also, cultivation was confirmed by archaeological evidence from the same period from the species retrieved from an Early Bronze Age layer at Sitagroi in Macedonia [7]. Coriander was used in two forms: as a spice for its seeds and as a herb for the flavor of its leaves for a long time, which was revealed from the Linear B tablets recovered from Pylos in which its' cultivation ismentioned for manufacturing of perfumes also [6].

ABOUT THE PLANT

It is a summer or winter cultivated annual crop. During the flowering stage, it can attain a height of 20- 140 cm. The plant has taproot and seeds germinate under epigeal type (rapid elongation of hypocotyl and upward arching). The plant stem is almost erect, sympodial, hollow, and monochasial-branched (3 branches at the basal node) with its basal parts (diameter up to 2 cm) (Figs. **1** and **2**) [8]. The inflorescence is present in each branch at ends. The color of the ribbed stem is green and sometimes turns to red or violet during the flowering period. The leaves are green or light green with shiny and waxy texture underside, decompounded, arranged alternately and often gathered in a rosette form. This diversifolius plant basal blade leaves are either undivided with three lobes or tripinnatifid. The higher degree of pinnatifidation is in nodal leaves. The upper leaves are deeply incised, with narrow lanceolate or even filiform-shaped blades [1, 8, 9], whereas the leaves on the lower region are stalked, short petioled, while the petiole of the upper leaves is reduced to a small, nearly amplexicaul (sessile with the base) leaf sheath. They are imparipinnate sect into linear- setaceous lobes.

The flowers are small, white or pinkish purple with compound terminal umbels. The compound umbel inflorescence has one or two linear bracts with 2-8 primary rays of different lengths with arranged umbellets. The umbellets with 5- 20 secondary rays are carried by two or more bracteoles. Initially, the flowering begins with the primary umbel having peripheral umbellets. The peripheral flowers first flowers in every umbellet [8, 9]. The flowers present at the center of umbellets are staminiferous or sometimes infertile. The five petals of the flowers outside the umbellets are lengthened and peripheral flowers are asymmetric. The flowers of the central region are circular and petals are bent inwards, while the petals are pale pink or white (Fig. **2c**).

The yellowish-brown ribbed fruits are globular or ovate, ribbed with a diameter of up to 6 mm. Usually, the schizocarp does not spontaneously split into two mericarps. The two mericarps have a sclerotized pericarp at the convex surface, while the pericarp in the concave is pellicular. In the center of the hollow fruits, a tiny carpophore is visible. Every mericarp has six longitudinal, straight side ribs on the convex outside, which is alternated with five waved, often hardly visible main ribs. On the convex inside, there are two longitudinal vittae, containing the essential oil of the ripe fruit. Starting from the root, there are schizogenic channels in all parts of the plant, which contain essential oils. These give the green plant a characteristic smell. This smell is caused by different aldehydic components of the essential oil present in the green plant. The ripe fruit has an inferior ovary with the five calyx teeth of different length surrounding the stylopodium (Fig. **2b**).

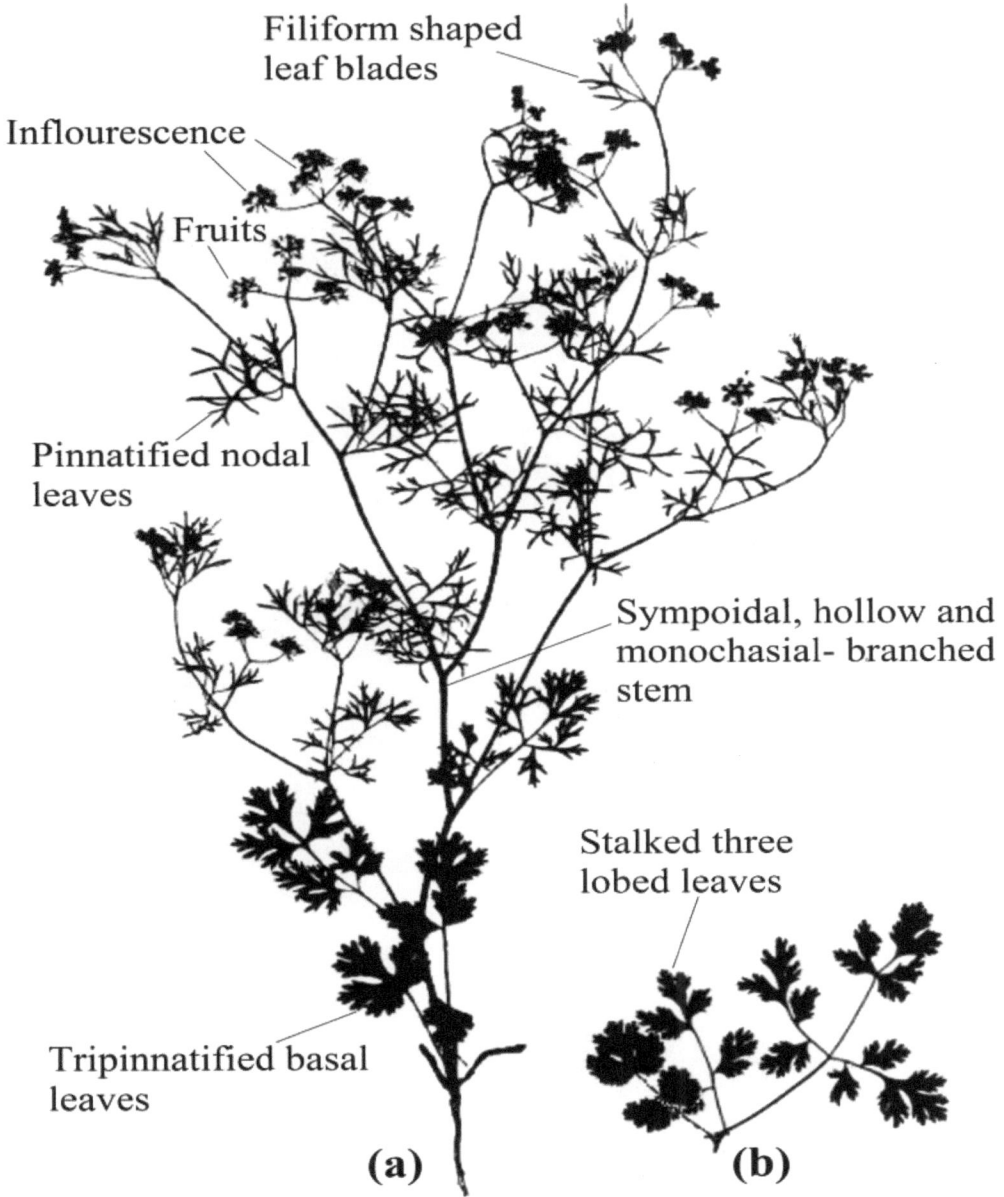

Fig. (1). (a) Flowering Coriander Plant (b) leaves of coriander [8].

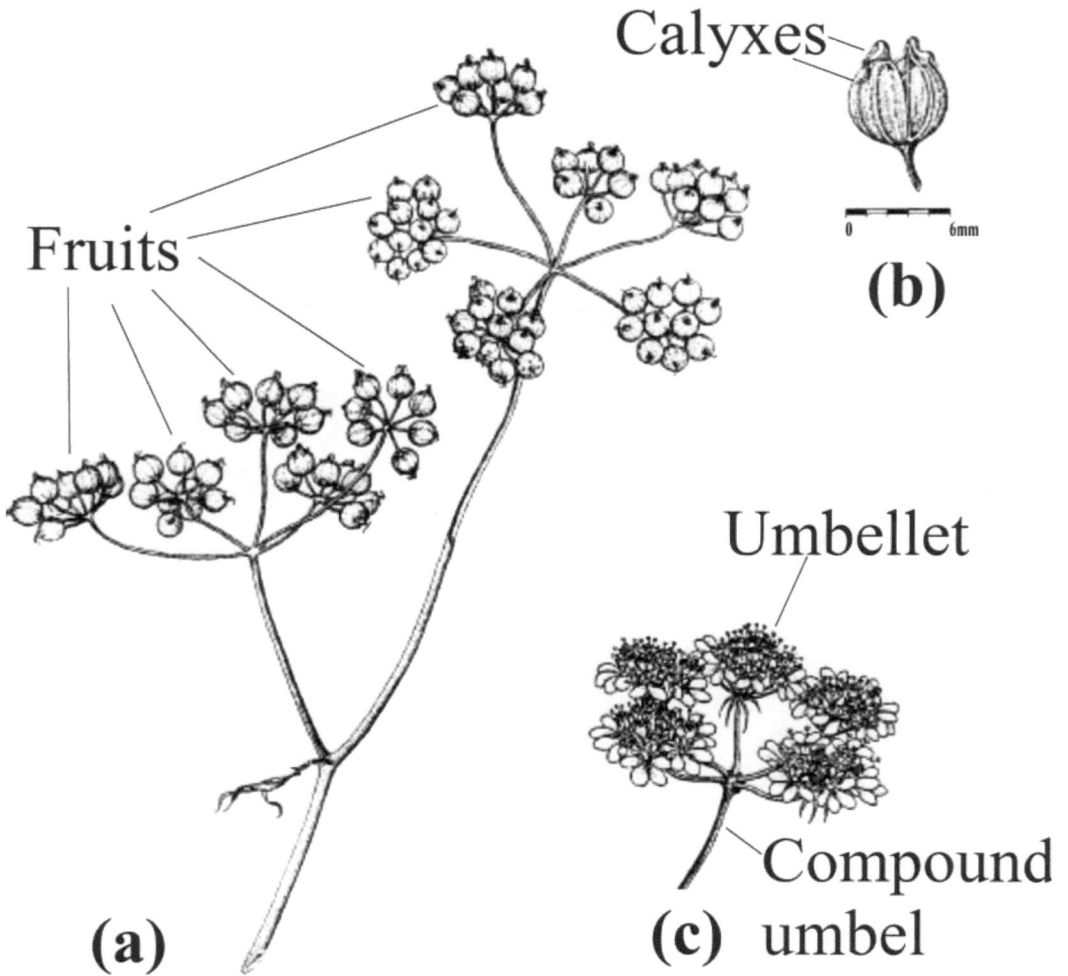

Fig. (2). (a) Branch of the ripe coriander fruits and **(b)** a fruit **(c)** Flowering branch of coriander [8].

Polygonal cells of epicarp have calcium oxalate crystals, whereas the central region of the mesocarp has fusiform sclerenchymatous tissues, which are arranged in sinuous rows. The outer 5 to 6 six rows of cells are arranged longitudinally and characteristically, the sinuous rows appeared as crossed right angles in the whole structure. Tracheids show bordered pits. The endocarp has an elongated single layer of lignified cells with thin walls. Endosperm is composed of aleurone grains and oil globules. Aseptate vittae with polygonal cells are arranged in two on the commissural surface, tapered at both ends (Fig. **3**)

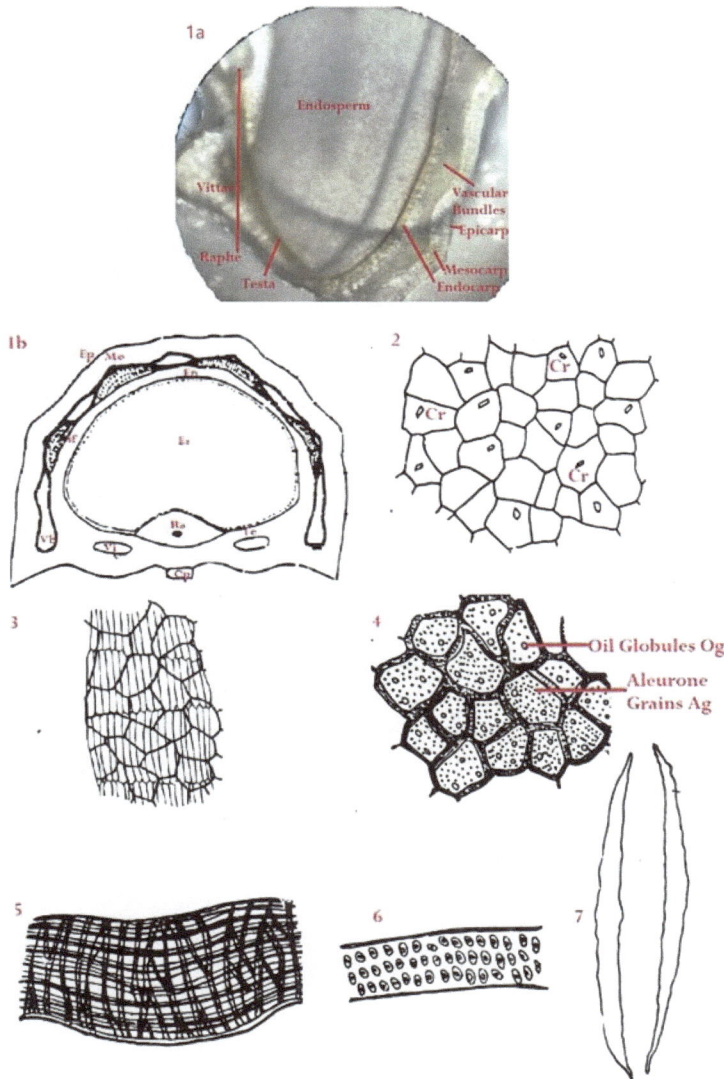

Fig. (3). Microscopic features of Coriander Fruit 1. T.S. of coriander mericarp 2. Epicarp in surface view 3. Rectangular sclereids of the mesocarp with underlying endocarp in view 4. Fragment of Endosperm 5. Sclerenchymatous tissue of Mesocarp 6. Tacheid showing bordered pits 7. Vittae. Here, Ag: Aleuronic grain; Cp: Carpophore; Cr: Crystal; En: Endocarp; Ep: Epicarp; Es: Endosperm; Me: Mesocarp; Og: Oil globule; Ra: Raphe; Sf: Sclerenchymatous fiber; Te: Testa; Vb: Vascular bundle; Vi: Vittae.

CHEMICAL CONSTITUENTS

The major constituent of the coriander is volatile oil (~1%) and linalool is the 60-70% part of it [9, 10]. The other constituents are monoterpene hydrocarbons (α-pinene, β- pinene, γ- terpinene, limonene, p- cymene, *etc.*; camphor, geraniol, borneol, citronellol, geranyl acetate); heterocyclic components, (pyrazine, furan, and tetrahydrofuran derivatives) [10, 11]; isocoumarins [12, 13], coriandrin and its ketonic derivatives A-E, dihydrocoriandrin; flavonoids; phthalide, z-digustilide and neochidilide [14]; phytosterols and phenolic acids.

During ripening, the aldehydic components disappear. Linalool is only present in the vittae of the fruits and it is not found in other parts of the plant. When completely ripe, only these vittae contain essential oil, while the additional channels in the mesocarp are flattened and disappear during ripening. During the ripening of the fruits, the aromatic properties of coriander changes drastically and the odor of the riped fruits are very different from that of the unripe fruits and the green herb.

PROPERTIES AND USES

The leaves of coriander are aromatic, acrid with analgesic, astringent, styptic, and anti-inflammatory activities. It is also useful in pharyngoplasty, chronic conjunctivitis, epistaxis, hiccup, halitosis, ulemorrhagia, inflammations, jaundice, odontalgia, hemorrhoids, and suppurations [9]. The fruits are aromatic, emollient, astringent, anti-inflammatory, thermogenic, stomachic, appetizer, stimulant, antipyretic, anodyne, and expectorant. In ayurvedic context, they are also useful in vitiated conditions of pitta, burning sensation, pharyngoplasty, cough, dyspepsia, bronchitis, vomiting, colic, flatulence, anorexia, dysentery, chronic conjunctivitis, diarrhea, cephalalgia, epistaxis, strangury, erysipelas, scrofula, hemorrhoids, edema, intermittent fevers, gout, hyperdipsia, giddiness, and rheumatism. A leaf paste is good for allergic inflammations caused by *Semecarpus anacardium* used historically to mark fabrics [1, 9].

TRADITIONAL USES

Traditionally, seeds of coriander are used as a diuretic in boiled water preparation with cumin in India. Seeds have also been used for anxiety and insomnia relief in Iran [15]. Holistically, it is used as a carminative, a general digestive aid [16, 17], anthelmintic, and inflammatory bowel diseases. Post-coital antifertility activity of seeds is also mentioned in a study [18].

PREPARATION & STORAGE

Coriander seeds are used coarsely or more finely powdered, as per the desired texture. Ground coriander loses its flavor and aroma quickly and should be stored in an opaque airtight container. The flavor of the seeds may be enhanced by a light roasting before use. In cooking, it can be used as a handful or a pinch as a spice [14]. Chopped leaves lose their flavor when dried, but may be frozen into ice cubes to preserve it.

PHYTOCHEMICAL INVESTIGATIONS

TLC Identity Test

The volatile oil, separated from the seeds by distillation, can be used for the identification by thin-layer chromatographic analysis. The sample of the oil is prepared in acetone, which is later chromatographed on pre-coated silica gel plates with toluene: ethyl acetate (93:7) as a solvent system. The spraying of vanillin sulphuric acid reagent helps in visualizing the pattern of oil components. The blue spot obtained in the chromatogram corresponds to the standard linalool (Retardation factor R_f 0.26). Other spots of the compounds can be confirmed with the respective standards.

Analysis of Volatile Oil

Various methods are used for determination and compound identification of essential oil of coriander, for example the oil was analyzed with GC-FID on two fused silica capillary columns (30 m × 0.2 mm i.d.) with bonded stationary phases: SPB-5 and SW-10 (Supelco, Switzerland), a film thickness of both columns was 0.25 µm. The carrier gas was helium with a split ratio of 1:150, and a flow rate of 20- 25 cm/sec. The injector temperature was 200°C and the oven temperature was programmed from 50 - 250°C, 2°C/min [19]. The individual components of the oil can be identified by their retention indices and compared with the standards from data banks or papers.

Eighteen components were reported to be ninety percent of the total volatile oil. Linalool is the most characteristic constituent of coriander oil. The other characteristic components of coriander oil are γ-terpinene (0.3 - 11.2%), α-pinene (0 - 10.9%), p-cymene (0.1 - 8.1%), camphor (1.2 - 5.3%), geranyl acetate (0.2 - 5.4%) and geraniol (0 - 3.6%). Limonene was found to be 0.1 - 3.2%, the other constituents were less than 1.5% of the total oil. The major component of the coriander's volatile oil, linalool, showed its presence at different concentrations, collected from different sources [20].

Limits for Quality Parameters

Some of the physicochemical parameters, which can be used as a quality control tool for coriander are: Foreign organic matter: No more than (NMT) 2.0% ; Total ash: NMT 6.0% ; Acid insoluble ash: NMT 1.0% ; Alcohol soluble extractive: No less than (NLT) 8.0% ; Water soluble extractive: NLT 16.0% ; Volatile oil: NLT 0.3% v/w [9].

PHARMACOLOGICAL INVESTIGATIONS

Diuretic Activity - The seeds of *Coriandrum sativum* L. Apiaceae had acute diuretic activity when a continuous intravenous infusion of an aqueous extract was administered in rats. It increased diuresis, excretion of electrolytes, and glomerular filtration rate in a dose-dependent manner like furosemide [21].

Anthelmintic Activity- Investigations on crude aqueous and hydro-alcoholic extracts of the seeds have shown anthelmintic activity on the egg and adult nematode parasite *Haemonchus contortus,* which was also confirmed to be present in sheep. The hydro-alcoholic extract has better in vitro activity against adult parasites than the aqueous one [22].

Antioxidant and Antibacterial Activity- The polyphenolic compounds of this spice have antioxidant potential when evaluated against hydrogen peroxide-induced oxidative damage in human lymphocytes. The total phenolic content of a methanolic and aqueous extract is high in freeze-dried and irradiated cilantro leaves and stems. *In vitro* studies have also supported these facts [23, 24]. In an investigation on leafy vegetables and their stored heated oil, coriander leaves have shown a protective effect on peroxide formation on the storage of heated oils, conferring them as excellent antioxidants that are stable at high temperatures and can serve as substitutes for synthetic antioxidants [25]. The aqueous extract with potential antioxidant effect has caffeic acid, protocatechuic acid, and glycitin in high concentration and in different fractions identifies gas chromatographically with a mass spectrophotometer. The β-carotene/linoleic acid model was similar to one another, but inferior to that of the crude extract and of butylated hydroxytoluene [26]. The seeds have stronger antioxidant activity than the leaves. The use of coriander in food products will increase the antioxidant content and as a natural antioxidant, inhibits unwanted oxidation processes [27]. The extract of coriander, prepared by supercritical extraction, produces odorless and tasteless antioxidant fractions with good activities [28].

Soil Degradation- Coriander generates a "soil degradation scent" as a volatile substance that affects the soil degradation by altering the physical, biological and chemical properties, and these need more scientific documentation [29].

Anxiolytic Activity- Aqueous extract of seed has anxiolytic effects evaluated in mice by an elevated plus-maze model. It reduces spontaneous activity and neuromuscular co-ordination. This suggests that coriander seeds may have potential sedative and muscle relaxant effects [30].

Antimutagenic Activity- Coriander juice has antimutagenic activity assessed by Ames reversion mutagenicity assay (his− to his+) with *S. typhimurium* TA98 strain as indicator organism on 4-nitro-o- phenylenediamine, m-phenylenediamine and 2-aminofluorene induced mutation [31].

Anti-inflammatory Activity- Coriander is also used as an anti-inflammatory agent in various polyherbal formulations, such as a formulation containing *Coriandrum sativum*, *Aegle marmeloes*, *Cyperus rotundus* and *Vetiveria zinzanioids,* showed significant inhibitory activity against inflammatory bowel disease [32]. It has various elements, including Cu, Zn, *etc.*, with varying concentrations when analyzed using X-ray fluorescence [33].

Antibacterial Activity- Gas chromatography Mass spectroscopic analysis (GCMS) of fractionally distilled components from volatile oil has shown the presence of long-chain (C6–C10) alcohols and aldehydes, which were active against gram-positive bacteria, gram-negative bacteria, and *Saccharomyces cerevisiae*. The essential oil of coriander was particularly effective against *Listeria monocytogenes* [34]. Coriander cells were metabolically competent and suitable for a plant cell microbe co-incubation assay, developed to analyze the promutagen activation by plant systems and can be used as an indicator of potential genetic effects [35].

Anti-implantation: Aqueous extract of fresh coriander seeds has anti-implantation effect. They produced a significant decrease in serum progesterone levels on day-5 of pregnancy in rats [18, 36].

Hypoglycemic Activity- Coriander seeds have significant hypoglycemic action as they have shown an increased concentration of hepatic glycogen from the increased activity of glycogen synthase [37].

Suppressive Activity on lead deposition- Chinese parsley, a coriander variety, has suppressive activity on the lead deposition, probably resulting from the chelation of lead by some substances [38].

CLINICAL INVESTIGATIONS

Coriander has been an integral part of traditional medicines as well as recipes in Asian countries and is prescribed for many ailments [39]. Although clinical investigations are restricted around therapeutic claims from traditional treaties, systematic evaluation of coriander beyond polyherbal formulations is still needed. The potential of coriander is reflected by some clinical trials, for example a randomized clinical trial study on 68 migraine patients treated with syrup of coriander fruit has shown that it reduces the duration and severity of migraine attacks by 50% as compared to the control group of patients. The study design included the effect of syrup on the duration, severity, and frequency of migraine for four weeks. Administration of 15 ml of syrup, three times per day, in patients already treated with sodium valproate (500 mg per day) was evaluated by recording migraine attacks per week, as well as their severity and duration [40]. Similarly, the effect of coriander fruits in combination with flowers of *Viola odorata* L. and *Rosa damascenea* L. for four-weeks, in 88 patients in the double-blinded, placebo-controlled design of a randomized clinical trial has shown the potential to effectively treat and reduce migraines. Patients under the study received this combination thrice a day and propranolol 20 mg twice a day for four weeks and compared with the control group (propranolol 20 mg treatment only). Clinical effects on duration and severity of migraines were then evaluated after completion of two and four-week treatment with the combination [41].

Coriander also has anti-inflammatory activity, which was investigated for periodontitis treatment in the form of a mucoadhesive gel. It comprises the extract of *Coriandrum sativum* fruit and seed hull of *Quercus brantii*, which was investigated in a randomized trial where 18 patients of chronic periodontitis and physicals were double-blinded. The gel was applied, as an adjuvant, twice during the observation period of three months. The variables evaluated for each patient were periodontal pocket depth, clinical attachment level, papilla bleeding index, and plaque index. The outcomes of the trial indicate significant improvement in periodontal indices [42]. In addition to this, coriander was also studied for diaper dermatitis. A non-randomized clinical trial on 58 infants was performed with a prescription of coriander gel and compared with hydrocortisone (1%) ointment. The treatment was offered for three days and applied twice daily to evaluate diaper dermatitis index and followed for 10 days. The outcomes of the study did not establish the efficacy of coriander gel in comparison to hydrocortisone; however, amendments in the formulation of gel and addition of soothing agents may improve the outcome in trials with a large sample [43]. Nonetheless, all these clinical studies suggest that coriander can be taken up for further clinical evaluations to validate and establish traditional claims associated with the pharmacological properties of coriander. It indicates a ray of hope that coriander could be developed as a key component of nutraceutical products for the treatment of various lifestyle-related disorders.

DISCUSSION

Humans have found that plants and herbs that are used to enhance the flavor of food can also help to restore health. Various phytochemical and pharmacological studies have been conducted to scientifically validate the traditional medicinal uses with their correlation to phytoconstituents present in different parts of the coriander. The review supported the potential of this spice as a medicinal plant.

The two parts of the plant, leaves and fruit, have more medicinal value and biologically active substances. The essential oil and different extracts from it have various pharmacological activities. The nutritional value of the fruit is also of paramount importance, which makes it usable as a spice and flavoring agent in food preparations.

CONCLUSION

It is now evident from several papers and investigation results that coriander is a classical and traditional remedy for various health disorders, including anxiety, sleeping disorders, insomnia, eye disorders, intermittent fever, hemorrhoids, rheumatism, dyspepsia, giddiness, post-coital antifertility activity, dysentery, epistaxis, halitosis, ulemorrhagia, pharyngoplasty, anorexia, and jaundice and it also works as a diuretic (a preparation of coriander and cumin seeds). Potential benefits of coriander in multiple domains establish its importance as a medicinal plant with food values.

CONSENT FOR PUBLICATION

Not applicable.

CONFLICT OF INTEREST

The authors confirm that there is no conflict of interest.

ACKNOWLEDGMENTS

Declared none.

REFERENCES

[1]   Sativum C. "Indian Medicinal Plants" (a compendium of 500 species). Orient Longman 2004; 2: 184.

[2]   "Coriander", Oxford English Dictionary. 2nd ed., Oxford University Press 1989.

[3]   Chadwick J. The Mycenaean World. Cambridge: University Press 1976; p. 119.

[4]   Zohary D, Hopf M. Domestication of plants in the Old World. 3rd ed. Oxford: University Press 2000; p. 206.

[5]   Akgul A. Baharat Bilimi ve Teknolojisi. Gıda Teknolojisi Derneg˘I Yayınları Yayın, Ankara 1993; 15:

113-4.

[6]   Aburjai T, Natsheh FM. Plants used in cosmetics. Phytother Res 2003; 17(9): 987-1000.
        [http://dx.doi.org/10.1002/ptr.1363] [PMID: 14595575]

[7]   Megaloudi F. Wild and cultivated vegetables, herbs and spices in greek antiquity (900 B.C. to 400
        B.C.). Environ Archaeol 2005; 10: 73-82.
        [http://dx.doi.org/10.1179/env.2005.10.1.73]

[8]   Diederichsen A. Promoting the conservation and use of underutilized and neglected crops. Coriander
        (*Coriandrum sativum* L.). International Plant Genetic Resources Institute (IPGRI), Rome 1996, pp.12-
        13.

[9]   Handa SS, Mundkinajeddu D, Joseph GVR. Indian Herbal Pharmacopoeia, vol. II. Regional Research
        Laboratory, Indian Drug Manufactures Association, (Eds.), 1999, pp. 9–16, 35–43.

[10]   Bisset NG. Herbal Drugs and Phytopharmaceuticals, Medpharm, Stittgart, (ed.), 1994, pp. 159.

[11]   Lamparsky D, Klinies I. Heterocyclic trace components in the essential oil of Coriander. Perfum
        Flavor 1988; 13-7.

[12]   Baba K, Xiao YQ, Taniguchi M, *et al.* Isocoumarins from *Coriandrum sativum*. Phytochemistry 1991;
        30: 4143.
        [http://dx.doi.org/10.1016/0031-9422(91)83482-Z]

[13]   Tanaguchi M, Yanai M, Xiao YQ, *et al.* Three isocoumarins from *Coriandrum sativum*.
        Phytochemistry 1996; 42: 843.
        [http://dx.doi.org/10.1016/0031-9422(95)00930-2]

[14]   Burdock GA, Carabin IG. Safety assessment of coriander (*Coriandrum sativum* L.) essential oil as a
        food ingredient. Food Chem Toxicol 2009; 47(1): 22-34.
        [http://dx.doi.org/10.1016/j.fct.2008.11.006] [PMID: 19032971]

[15]   Ganesan P, Phaiphan A, Murugan Y, Baharin BS. Comparativestudy of bioactive compounds in curry
        and coriander leaves: an update. J Chem Pharm Res 2013; 5: 590-4.

[16]   Burdock GA, Carabin IG. Safety assessment of coriander (*Coriandrum sativum* L.) essential oil as a
        food ingredient. Food Chem Toxicol 2009; 47(1): 22-34.
        [http://dx.doi.org/10.1016/j.fct.2008.11.006] [PMID: 19032971]

[17]   Ravi R, Prakash M, Bhat KK. Aroma characterization of coriander (*Coriandrum sativum* L.) oil
        samples. Eur Food Res Technol 2007; 225: 367-74.
        [http://dx.doi.org/10.1007/s00217-006-0425-7]

[18]   Al-Said MS, Al-Khamis KI, Islam MW, Parmar NS, Tariq M, Ageel AM. Post-coital antifertility
        activity of the seeds of *Coriandrum sativum* in rats. J Ethnopharmacol 1987; 21(2): 165-73.
        [http://dx.doi.org/10.1016/0378-8741(87)90126-7] [PMID: 3437767]

[19]   Orav A, Arak E, Raal A. Essential Oil Composition of *Coriandrum sativum* L. Fruits from Different
        Countries. JOEB 2011; 14: 118-23.

[20]   Msaada K, Hosni K, Ben Taarit M, *et al.* Variations in essential oil composition during maturation of
        coriander (*Coriandrum sativum* L.) fruits. J Food Chem 2009; 33: 603-12.
        [http://dx.doi.org/10.1111/j.1745-4514.2009.00240.x]

[21]   Aissaoui A, El-Hilaly J, Israili ZH, Lyoussi B. Acute diuretic effect of continuous intravenous infusion
        of an aqueous extract of *Coriandrum sativum* L. in anesthetized rats. J Ethnopharmacol 2008; 115(1):
        89-95.
        [http://dx.doi.org/10.1016/j.jep.2007.09.007] [PMID: 17961943]

[22]   Eguale T, Tilahun G, Debella A, Feleke A, Makonnen E. *In vitro* and *in vivo* anthelmintic activity of
        crude extracts of *Coriandrum sativum* against *Haemonchus contortus*. J Ethnopharmacol 2007; 110(3):
        428-33.
        [http://dx.doi.org/10.1016/j.jep.2006.10.003] [PMID: 17113738]

[23] Peter WYY, David KD. Studies on the dual antioxidant and antibacterial properties of parsley *(Petroselinum crispum)* and cilantro (*Coriandrum sativum*) extracts. Food Chem 2006; 97: 505-15. [http://dx.doi.org/10.1016/j.foodchem.2005.05.031]

[24] Hashim MS, Lincy S, Remya V, *et al.* Effect of polyphenolic compounds from *Coriandrum sativum* on H_2O_2-induced oxidative stress in human lymphocytes. Food Chem 2005; 92: 653-60. [http://dx.doi.org/10.1016/j.foodchem.2004.08.027]

[25] Shyamala BN, Gupta S, Jyothi L, *et al.* Leafy vegetable extracts—antioxidant activity and effect on storage stability of heated oils. Innov Food Sci Emerg Technol 2005; 6: 239-45. [http://dx.doi.org/10.1016/j.ifset.2004.12.002]

[26] Melo EDA, Filho JM, Guerra NB. Characterization of antioxidant compounds in aqueous coriander extract *(Coriandrum sativum* L.). Lebensm Wiss Technol 2005; 38: 15-9. [http://dx.doi.org/10.1016/j.lwt.2004.03.011]

[27] Wangensteen H, Samuelsen AB, Malterud KE. Antioxidant activity in extracts from coriander. Food Chem 2004; 88: 293-7. [http://dx.doi.org/10.1016/j.foodchem.2004.01.047]

[28] Yepez B, Espinos M, Lopez S, *et al.* Producing antioxidant fractions from herbaceous matrices by supercritical fluid extraction. Fluid Phase Equilib 2002; 2: 879-84. [http://dx.doi.org/10.1016/S0378-3812(01)00707-5]

[29] Fuente EDL, Lenardis AE, Suárez SA, *et al.* Insect communities related to wheat and coriander cropping histories and essential oils in the Rolling Pampa, Argentina. Eur J Agron 2006; 24: 385-95. [http://dx.doi.org/10.1016/j.eja.2006.01.004]

[30] Emamghoreishi M, Khasaki M, Aazam MF. *Coriandrum sativum*: evaluation of its anxiolytic effect in the elevated plus-maze. J Ethnopharmacol 2005; 96(3): 365-70. [http://dx.doi.org/10.1016/j.jep.2004.06.022] [PMID: 15619553]

[31] Cortés-Eslava J, Gómez-Arroyo S, Villalobos-Pietrini R, Espinosa-Aguirre JJ. Antimutagenicity of coriander (*Coriandrum sativum*) juice on the mutagenesis produced by plant metabolites of aromatic amines. Toxicol Lett 2004; 153(2): 283-92. [http://dx.doi.org/10.1016/j.toxlet.2004.05.011] [PMID: 15451560]

[32] Jagtap AG, Shirke SS, Phadke AS. Effect of polyherbal formulation on experimental models of inflammatory bowel diseases. J Ethnopharmacol 2004; 90(2-3): 195-204. [http://dx.doi.org/10.1016/j.jep.2003.09.042] [PMID: 15013181]

[33] Al-Bataina BA, Maslat AO, Al-Kofahil MM. Element analysis and biological studies on ten oriental spices using XRF and Ames test. J Trace Elem Med Biol 2003; 17(2): 85-90. [http://dx.doi.org/10.1016/S0946-672X(03)80003-2] [PMID: 14531636]

[34] Delaquis PJ, Stanich K, Girard B, Mazza G. Antimicrobial activity of individual and mixed fractions of dill, cilantro, coriander and eucalyptus essential oils. Int J Food Microbiol 2002; 74(1-2): 101-9. [http://dx.doi.org/10.1016/S0168-1605(01)00734-6] [PMID: 11929164]

[35] Cortés-Eslava J, Gómez-Arroyo S, Villalobos-Pietrini R, Espinosa-Aguirre JJ. Metabolic activation of three arylamines and two organophosphorus insecticides by coriander (*Coriandrum sativum*) a common edible vegetable. Toxicol Lett 2001; 125(1-3): 39-49. [http://dx.doi.org/10.1016/S0378-4274(01)00414-3] [PMID: 11701221]

[36] Vasudeva N, Sharma SK. Post-coital antifertility activity of Achyranthes aspera Linn. root. J Ethnopharmacol 2006; 107(2): 179-81. [http://dx.doi.org/10.1016/j.jep.2006.03.009] [PMID: 16725289]

[37] Chithra V, Leelamma S. *Coriandrum sativum* — mechanism of hypoglycemic action. Food Chem 1999; 67: 229-31. [http://dx.doi.org/10.1016/S0308-8146(99)00113-2]

[38] Aga M, Iwaki K, Ueda Y, *et al.* Preventive effect of *Coriandrum sativum* (Chinese parsley) on localized lead deposition in ICR mice. J Ethnopharmacol 2001; 77(2-3): 203-8.
[http://dx.doi.org/10.1016/S0378-8741(01)00299-9] [PMID: 11535365]

[39] Ibn-e-Sina AH, Fit-tib Al-Qanun. The Canon of Medicine (research of ebrahim shamsedine). Beirut, Lebanon: Alaalami Beirut library Press 2005.

[40] Delavar Kasmaei H, Ghorbanifar Z, Zayeri F, *et al.* Effects of *Coriandrum sativum* Syrup on Migraine: A Randomized, Triple-Blind, Placebo-Controlled Trial. Iran Red Crescent Med J 2016; 18(1)e20759
[http://dx.doi.org/10.5812/ircmj.20759] [PMID: 26889386]

[41] Kamali M, Seifadini R, Kamali H, Mehrabani M, Jahani Y, Tajadini H. Efficacy of combination of Viola odorata, Rosa damascena and *Coriandrum sativum* in prevention of migraine attacks: a randomized, double blind, placebo-controlled clinical trial. Electron Physician 2018; 10(3): 6430-8.
[http://dx.doi.org/10.19082/6430] [PMID: 29765566]

[42] Yaghini J, Shahabooei M, Aslani A, Zadeh MR, Kiani S, Naghsh N. Efficacy of a local-drug delivery gel containing extracts of *Quercus brantii* and *Coriandrum sativum* as an adjunct to scaling and root planing in moderate chronic periodontitis patients. J Res Pharm Pract 2014; 3(2): 67-71.
[http://dx.doi.org/10.4103/2279-042X.137076] [PMID: 25114940]

[43] Dastgheib L, Pishva N, Saki N, *et al.* SEfficacy of topical *Coriandrum sativum* extract on treatment of infants with diaper dermatitis: a single blinded non-randomised controlled trial. Malays J Med Sci 2017; 24(4): 97-101.
[http://dx.doi.org/10.21315/mjms2017.24.4.11] [PMID: 28951694]

CHAPTER 8

Flax Seed (*Linum usitatissimum*): a Potential Functional Food Source

Vishal Soni and **Priyanka Soni**

Department of Pharmacognosy, B. R. Nahata College of Pharmacy, Mandsaur, M.P., India

Abstract: Flax (*Linum usitatissimum*), from the family Linaceae, is a blue blossoming yearly spice that produces shorts seeds fluctuating from golden yellow to ruddy earthy colored shading. Flaxseed has a fresh surface and nutty taste. Flaxseed oil is believed to bring mental and physical perseverance by battling weariness and controlling the maturing procedure. Flaxseed is rich in dietary dissolvable and insoluble strands. other">Because of its high substance of lignans, it plays an important role in the reduction of joint inflammation, hypercholesterolemia, atherosclerosis, other">phytoestrogens malady, malignant growth, hypertension, diabetes, other">osteoporosis, and neurological issues. Flaxseed has also been reported to act as anti-arrhythmic, anti-atherogenic, and improving the vascular functions. Among the useful nourishments, flaxseed has risen as a potential utilitarian food containing alpha-linolenic acid, lignans, great protein, and soluble fiber. Flaxseed cotyledons are the significant oil stockpiling tissues, containing 75% of the seed oil. Flaxseed oil contains 98% triacylglycerol, phospholipids, and 0.1% free unsaturated fats. Flaxseeds also contain a decent measure of phenolic mixes. It fills in a decent amount of minerals particularly, phosphorous (650 mg/100 g), magnesium (350–431 mg/100 g), calcium (236–250 mg/100 g), and has an exceptionally low measure of sodium (27 mg/100 g). It is also associated with the supplementation of Omega-3 polyunsaturated fatty acids. Flaxseeds have various biological and pharmacological effects like anti-diabetic, cancer reducing effects, hypocholesterolemic and cardiovascular diseases, prevention of kidney diseases, prevention and treatment of obesity, irritable bowel syndrome anti-thrombotic, *etc*.

Different clinical preliminaries revealed that flaxseed constituents give infection preventive and restorative advantages. More *in vivo* examinations are required to determine the medical advantages of flaxseed constituents. To know its remedial potential for all populace, including pregnant and lactating ladies and to realize potential issues associated with its overdose, a study needs to be carried out. There is a requirement for the advancement of fast, reproducible, and financial procedures for the examination of nutraceuticals from flaxseed.

---

* **Corresponding author Priyanka Soni**: B.R. Nahata College of Pharmacy, Mandsaur, M.P., India; Tel: 9993346486; E-mail: soni_priyanka21@rediffmail.com

Atta-ur-Rahman, M. Iqbal Choudhary & Sammer Yousuf (Eds.)

Cleaning the flaxseed ought to be viewed as a significant advance in decreasing the microbial tallies. Impacts of cleaning flaxseed on microbial burdens including aerobic plate counts (APCs), mold counts (MCs) yeast counts (YCs), coliform counts (CCs), *Escherichia coli* counts, and Enterobacteriaceae counts (ECs) were resolved. Flaxseeds contain enemies of supplements that may have an antagonistic impact on the wellbeing and prosperity of the human populace.Cyanogenic glycosides are the significant enemies of supplements in the digestive system. cyanogenic glycosides discharge hydrogen cyanide, a powerful respiratory inhibitor, by intestinal β-glycosidase that produces thiocyanates. Thiocyanates meddle with iodine take-up by the thyroid organ and create iodine-insufficiency issues, goiter, and cretinism. In this survey, supplements, useful properties, digestion, and medical advantages of bioactive particles viz., basic unsaturated fats, lignans, and dietary fiber of flaxseed will be discussed.

Keywords: Anti-nutrients, Anti-oxidants, Anti-arrhythmic, Anti-atherogenic and anti-inflammatory agent, Dietary fibers, Flaxseed, Flax (*Linum usitassimum*), Functional food, Lineaceae.

INTRODUCTION

Flaxseed is probably the most the oldest crop, cultivated the beginning of The Latin name of the flaxseed is *Linum usitatissimum*, which signifies "valuable [1]. Flax (*Linum usitassimum*) having a family Lineaceae, is a blue blooming yearly spice that produces little level seeds. Flaxseed is otherwise called linseed and these terms are utilized conversely. Fluctuating from brilliant yellow to rosy earthy colored shading. Flaxseed has a fresh surface and nutty taste [2].In the most recent two decades, flaxseed has been the focal point of expanded enthusiasm for the field of diet and malady research because of the potential medical advantages related to a portion of its organically dynamic parts [3]. Flaxseeds have dietary attributes and are a rich wellspring of ω-3 unsaturated fat: α-linolenic acid (ALA), short-chain polyunsaturated unsaturated fats (PUFA), solvent and insoluble strands, phytoestrogenic lignans (secoisolariciresinol diglucoside-SDG), proteins, and a variety of cancer prevention agents [4, 5]. Its developing ubiquity is because of wellbeing granting benefits in diminishing cardiovascular infections, diminished danger of malignant growth, especially of the mammary and prostate organ, calming movement, diuretic impact, and mitigation of menopausal side effects and osteoporosis. Flaxseed has been delegated a utilitarian food since it gives various medical advantages notwithstanding filling in as a wellspring of supplements [6]. Seeds are oval lenticular 4-6 mm long. The seed surface is smooth sparkling and dull earthy colored. They are slightly flattened and have one edge more acute than the other. Indian linseeds are classified into broad types for commercial purposes, namely, yellow and brown. Both the varieties are with almost similar nutritional values, but the yellow variety is preferable to the brown type, because of the higher percentage and lighter color of oil [7].

Occurrence and Distribution

The flax plant is a native of Egypt. It is unknown in a wild state and its origin is uncertain. Some consider it to be indigenous to localities between the Persian Gulf and the Caspian and Black seas, while others ascribe its origin to India. These two main geographical groups correspond to the oldest areas of cultivation. The important flaxseed growing countries include India, China, the United States, and Ethiopia. India is a leading country for the production of flaxseed. It is cultivated in different states namely, Madhya Pradesh, Maharashtra, Chhattisgarh, and Bihar [8]. The mature flaxseed is oblong and flattened, and having shiny yellow to dark brown seed coat (hull) (Fig. **1**) [9].

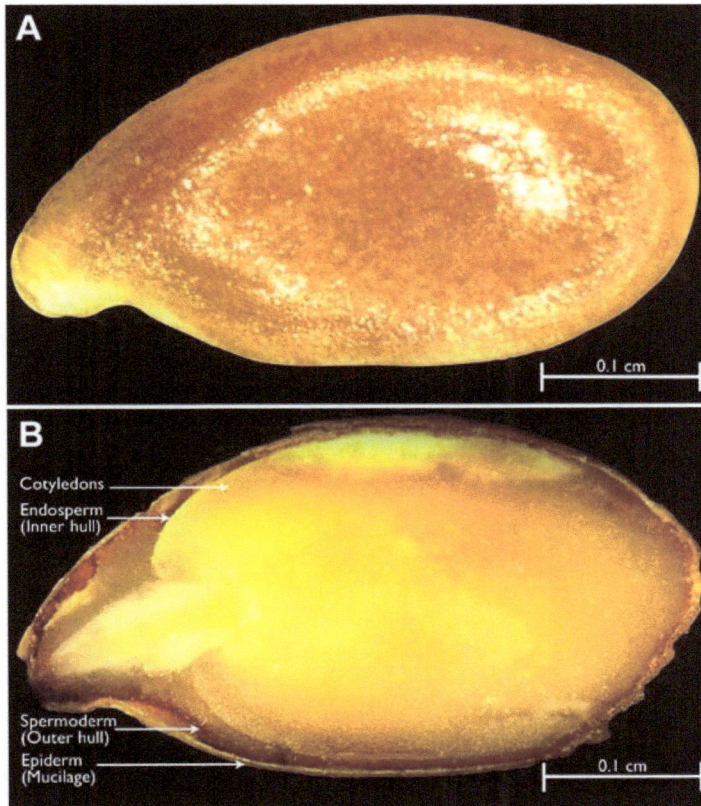

Fig. (1). Hand-cut sections of flaxseed (L. usitatissimum L., var. CDC Bethune) mounted in distilled water showing anatomical structures. **(A)** The side of the flaxseed **(B)** Hand-cut section of flaxseed [10].

Flax (*Linum usitassimum*) is a blue flowering annual herb that produces small flat seeds varying from golden yellow to reddish-brown color. Flaxseed possesses a crispy texture and nutty taste (Fig. **2**).

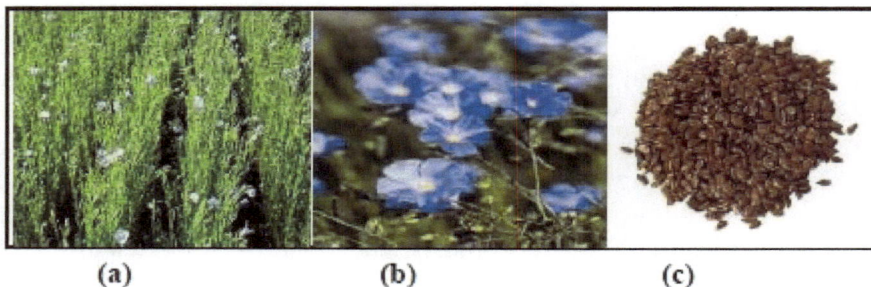

(a)   (b)   (c)

Fig. (2). Photograph of *Linum usitatissimum a)* Plant b) Flower c) Seeds [10].

TRADITION AND ETHANOMEDICAL USE

The flaxseed oil has the following medicinal properties:

- Maintain the skin pH
- Recovers tensile strength of the skin
- Increases moisture-holding capacity of the skin
- Wound healing
- Antitumor activity
- Anti-inflammatory
- Hepatoprotective activity [11].

Among the functional foods, flaxseed has emerged as a potential functional food is a good source of alpha-linolenic acid, lignans, high-quality protein, soluble fiber, and phenolic compounds. The composition of flaxseed is presented in Table **1**.

PHYTOCHEMICALS

Nutrients Composition of Flaxseed and Health Benefits

The flaxseeds are rich sources of secondary metabolites like α-linolenic acid (ALA), lignans, protein, dietary fiber, soluble polysaccharides, phenolic compounds, vitamins, and mineral [14, 54]. The chemical composition of nutrient and phytochemicals in flaxseed are shown in Table **2**.

Table 1. Traditional and medicinal uses of flaxseeds in various health problems [12, 13, 52].

Flax Form Consumed	Preparation/Processing Method	Traditional/Medicinal Health Benefits
Flaxseed tea	Uncrushed flaxseeds are soaked in water for 30 min. Seeds are then removed while the water is warmed moderately	• Useful against dyspnoea, asthma, dysphonia, bad cough, and bronchitis
Flaxseed drink	A teaspoon of flaxseed powder is put into a glass of hot water, brewed and drained. A cup of this water is to be taken daily.	• Helps out constipation
Flaxseed flour	Flaxseed flour 10-gram each for the concerned ailment is given a paste-like consistency using honey, 30-40 g of this paste is swallowed on an empty stomach in the morning.	• Used against pulmonary tuberculosis, haemoptysis, splenomegaly, and stomach ulcer. Cures inflammations of intestines and abdominal pains. • Disinfects gastrointestinal tract. • Strengthens the nervous system. • Strengthens the memory. • Good in treating the impairment of concentration. • Good in the management of age-associated distractibility. • Ensures rapid healing of wounds through external use. • Protects the skin against getting dry. • Used in eczema and psoriasis diseases. • Exercises a positive impact on respiratory tract diseases. • Good in curing mental disorders.

Proteins

The protein substance of flaxseed changes from 20 to 30%, comprising around 80% globulins (linen and conlinin) and 20% glutelin. It additionally contains peptides with bioactivities identified with the decline in chance components of CVD.

Dietary Fibers

Flax strands are among the most established fiber crops on the planet. Flax strands are separated from the skin of the stem of the plant. The complete flax plant is roughly 25% seed and 75% stem and leaves. The stem or non-seed parts are around 20% fiber, which can be removed by concoction or mechanical retting. Flax fiber is a characteristic and biodegradable composite, which displays great mechanical properties and low thickness. Plant lignans are phenolic mixes framed by the association of two cinnamic corrosive buildups. Lignans go about as the two cancer prevention agents and phytoestrogens. Phytoestrogens can have powerless estrogen movement in creatures and people [17].

Table 2. Chemical composition of nutrient and phytochemicals in flaxseed [15, 16].

Nutrients Amount Per 100 g of Edible Flaxseed	Nutrients Amount Per 100 g of Edible Flaxseed
Moisture (g) 6.5	Protein (N×6.25) (g) 20.3
Fat (g) 37.1	Minerals (g) 2.4
Crude fiber (g) 4.8	Total dietary fiber (g) 24.5
Carbohydrates (g) 28.9	Energy (kcal) 530.0
Potassium 750.0	Calcium (mg) 170.0
Phosphorous (mg) 370.0	Iron (mg) 2.7
Vitamin A (μg) 30.0	Vitamin E (mg) 0.6
Thiamine (B1) (mg) 0.23	Riboflavin (B2) (mg) 0.07
Niacin (mg) 1.0	Pyridoxine (mg) 0.61
Pantothenic acid 0.57	Biotin (μg) 0.6
Folic acid (μg) 112	
Moisture (g) 6.5	Protein (N×6.25) (g) 20.3
Fat (g) 37.1	Minerals (g) 2.4
Crude fiber (g) 4.8	Total dietary fiber (g) 24.5
Carbohydrates (g) 28.9	Energy (kcal) 530.0
Potassium 750.0	Calcium (mg) 170.0
Phosphorous (mg) 370.0	Iron (mg) 2.7
Vitamin A (μg) 30.0	Vitamin E (mg) 0.6
Thiamine (B1) (mg) 0.23	Riboflavin (B2) (mg) 0.07
Niacin (mg) 1.0	Pyridoxine (mg) 0.61
Pantothenic acid 0.57	Biotin (μg) 0.6
Biotin (μg) 0.6	Folic acid (μg) 112
Biotin (μg) 0.6	Folic acid (μg) 112

Minerals

Concerning the composition of minerals, the contents of calcium, magnesium, and phosphorus are highlighted being that a 30 g portion of the seed constitutes 7% to 30% of the recommended dietary allowances (RDAs) for these minerals.

Lignans

Lignans are phytoestrogens, which are abundantly available in fiber-rich plants, cereals (wheat, barley, and oats), legumes (bean, lentil, and soybean), vegetables (broccoli, garlic, asparagus, carrots) fruits, berries, tea, and alcoholic beverages. Flaxseed contains about 75–800 times more lignans than cereal grains, legumes, fruits, and vegetables [18].

Flaxseed Oil/Lipids

Flaxseed containing a higher amount of the ω-3 fatty acid *i.e.* α- linolenic acid [19, 20].

Bioactive Compounds

The phenolics, lignans, selenium, and cyclolino peptides were isolated from the flaxseeds, structure shown in Fig. (**3**).

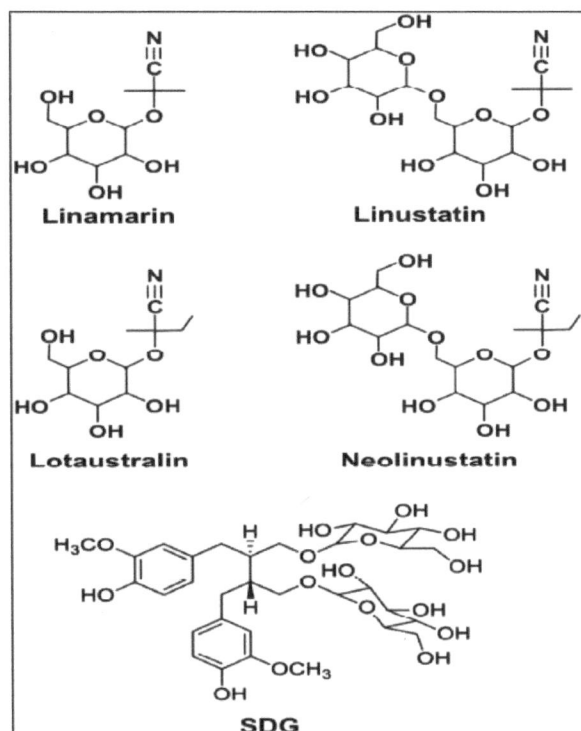

Fig. (3). Structures of four cyanogenic glycosides (mono-glycosides: linamarin, lotaustralin; di-glycosides: linustatin and neolinustatin) and SDG in flaxseed [21].

Flaxseed contains biologically active estrogenic compounds called phytoestrogens which helps in decreasing cell proliferation and prevents cancer. Higher levels of flaxseed are associated with the prevention of memory loss and constipation. Flaxseed also contains several non-nutritional compounds such as cyanogenic glycosides, cadmium, trypsin inhibitors, and phytic acid that negatively influence health and well-being. Fig. **4** shows a bioactive compound isolated from different parts of *Linum usitatissimum*.

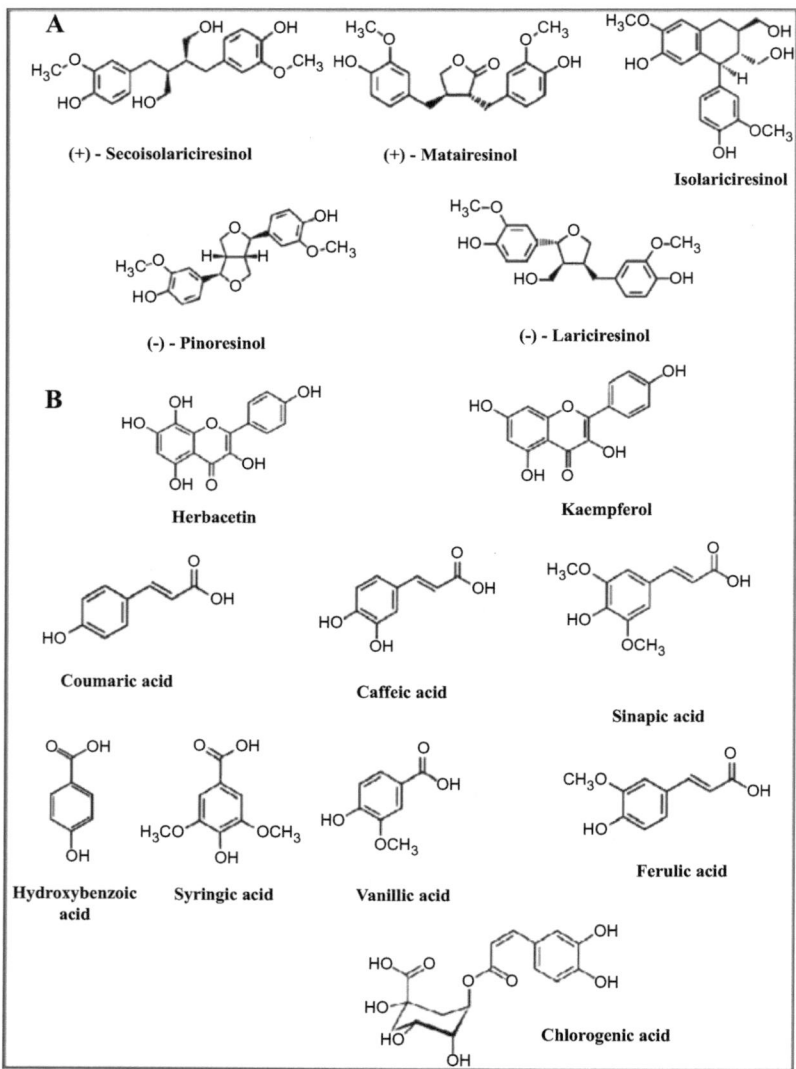

Fig. (4). Bioactive compound isolated from different parts of *Linum usitatissimum* [22, 23].

PHARMACOLOGICAL ACTION

Scientific literature and various actions have been reported to possess by *Linum usitatissimum.* Some pharmacological actions and therapeutic uses are as follows: The seeds are tonic, aphrodisiac, resolvent, antitussive, antilipidemic, laxative, demulcent, expectorant, diuretics, emollient, galactagogue, and emmenagogue. Roasted seeds are astringent Linseed poultice is emollient. Flowers are cardiac and nervine tonic [24].

Anti-Inflammatory

The anti-inflammatory activity of flaxseed oil was documented against carrageenan and prostaglandin E2(PGE2) induced paw edema in rats. The findings demonstrated significant anti-inflammatory activity by inhibiting the COX-II [25].

Antimicrobial

The oil of flaxseeds showed prominent antibacterial activity against *Salmonella typhi, Enterococcus, Escherichia coli, Bacillus subtilis,* and *Staphylococcus aureus* [26].

Antioxidant

The different models of antioxidant activity namely DPPH radical, reducing power, superoxide anion radical scavenging, hydroxyl radical scavenging, metal chelating, and hydrogen peroxide scavenging by EE-LU and α-tocopherol demonstrated significant antioxidant activity [27].

Antipyretic

The oil has antipyretic activity by reducing the temperature of the rats, and activity was comparable to aspirin [28].

Anti-Ulcer

The flaxseed oil reported the significant antiulcer activity against ethanol-induced gastric ulcers.

Laxative

The flaxseed has higher swelling index property and due to this, it produces laxative activity [29].

Bone Development

Flaxseed, in particular lignans, could influence bone development. In a study rats exposed to 88 or 177.3 mg SDG/kg of body weight/day had higher bone strength than the basal diet at 50 days post-natal. However, by post-natal day132, no differences in bone strength, bone mineral density were observed. Exposure to SDG did not have a negative effect on bone strength [30].

Hair Growth

The flaxseed increases the growth of hair length and also has a positive effect on hair density.

Atherosclerosis

Flaxseeds reduce the oxidative stress and control the production of cholesterol and decrease the serum level of HDL-C. This represents significant atherosclerosis and lowering the relative risk of coronary artery disease [31].

Memory

Loss in spatial memory is very much associated with the accumulation of lipid peroxide in the hippocampus. Higher levels of flaxseed nutritional, as well as non-nutritional components like antioxidants in the form N-3 fatty acids most often referred to as ω-3 fatty acids *i.e.* ALA, docosahexaenoic acid (DHA), and dietary fibers *i.e.* lignans, in addition to the reduction of body mass, reduces levels of lipid peroxide in the hippocampus. Studies on flax feed dam suggest that improvement in hippocampus ALA and DHA concentration results in the reduction of spatial memory inhibitors thus increases the learning ability of flaxseed feed dams [32].

Cardiovascular Diseases

Eicosanoids derived from omega-3-fatty acids, present in flaxseed primarily improves heart function by reducing blood cholesterol. A proportionate effect on blood cholesterol concentration and low-density lipoprotein fraction has been linked with higher concentrations of flaxseeds in the diets indicating a greater reduction in LDL protein, serum, and liver cholesterol [33, 34].

Blood Pressure

ω-3 fatty acids present in flaxseed have been found to regulate transcription and expression of genes, thereby altering enzyme synthesis and modifying several risk factors for coronary heart diseases, including reducing serum triglycerides and blood pressure [35].

Breast Cancer

The experimental rat treated with the flaxseed reduces the size and number of breast tumors [36, 37].

Prostate Cancer

The flaxseed has tumor-suppressive properties due to the influence of lignans [38].

Diabetes

The administration of flaxseed as a dietary supplement reduces the glucose level in blood due to the presence of fibers, lignans, and ω-3 fatty acids. Further, it also acts as an antiobesity agent [39, 40].

Kidney Diseases

The ω-3 fatty acids present in seeds can protect the kidney of old age patients and exhibited significant nephroprotective activity [41].

CLINICAL AND PRECLINICAL STUDIES (TABLE 3)

Table 3. Recent clinical reports showing lipid profile and other health effects of flaxseed consumption in the diet [42 - 44].

Experiment	Model System	Significant Findings	References
Consumption of 5 g of flax fibers daily for 1 week in the form of bread and drinks	Young healthy adults	Fecal excretion of fat increased by 50%. Flax bread and Flax drink reduced the Total & the LDL-cholesterol by 7 & 9 and 12 & 15%, respectively.	Kristensen *et al.* (2012)
Consumption of 5 g of flaxseed gums per day for 3 months	Type-2 diabetics	Total and LDL-cholesterol were reduced by 10 and 16%, respectively.	Thakur *et al.* (2009)
15% flaxseed meal enriched biscuits were fed for 8 weeks	Hypercholesterolemic rats	Cholesterol & triglyceride level decreased from 456.66 & 173.84 to 183.92 & 102.67 mg/dl,respectively. LDL and VLDL decreased from 199.46 & 34.95 to 84.08 & 20.53 mg/dl, respectively. While, HDL increased from 38.95 to 64.37 mg/dl.	Hassan *et al.* (2012)

(Table 3) cont.....

Experiment	Model System	Significant Findings	References
100% flaxseed oil was used as shortening in preparation of biscuits, which were fed for 8 weeks	Hypercholesterolemic rats	Cholesterol & triglyceride level decreased from 456.66 & 173.84 to 170.48 & 96.79 mg/dl, respectively. LDL and VLDL decreased from 199.46 & 34.95 to 74.79 & 19.34 mg/dl, respectively. While, HDL increased from 38.95 to 66.09 mg/dl.	Hassan *et al.* (2012)
Flaxseeds were consumed to see its effect on appetite-regulating hormones; lipemia and glycemia.	Young men	Decreased triglyceride levels (postprandial lipemia), Higher mean-ratings of satiety and fullness.	Kristensen *et al.* (2011)
Flaxseed powder enriched diets were consumed for 12-weeks to check body weight and lipid profile	Rats	Rats fed with high fat & high fructose diet along with 0.02% flax powder showed decreased levels of TG, total cholesterol, and LDL-cholesterol from 100, 69, and 10 to 96, 63 and 9 mg/dl, respectively.	Park and Velasquez (2012)
Animals were fed with 10%, 20% & 30% of raw and heated flaxseed in the basal diet for 30 days	Rats	Total cholesterol level got significantly reduced in all flaxseed groups and HDL- cholesterol got significantly increased by 20% raw; 30% raw and heated flaxseed groups. A significant reduction in LDL-cholesterol level was only observed in 30% raw flaxseed groups.	Khalesi *et al.* (2011)
Diets containing 2·7% flaxseed, 4·5% fiber and 3·7% ALA were fed for 10 weeks.	Mice	The median number of adenomas in the small intestine was 54 & 37 for control & flaxseed groups, respectively. Compared with controls(1·2 mm), the adenoma size was smaller in the flaxseed (0·9 mm) fed group.	Oikarinen *et al.* (2005)
Diets containing 2·7% flaxseed, 4·5% fiber and 3·7% ALA were fed for 10 weeks	Mice	The median number of adenomas in the small intestine was 54 & 37 for control & flaxseed groups, respectively. Compared with controls (1·2 mm), the adenoma size was smaller in the flaxseed (0·9 mm) fed group.	Oikarinen *et al.* (2005)
Animals were fed the basal diet (control) and ω-3 rich flax cotyledon's fraction (82 g/kg), respectively for 8 weeks	Mice	Flax diet reduced the cell proliferation; suppressed insulin growth factor (IGF)-1R and the growth of breast tumor.	Chen *et al.* (2011a, b)

(Table 3) cont.....

Experiment	Model System	Significant Findings	References
Isoenergetic diets were consumed for 28 days each containing approximately 36% energy from fat, of which 70% was provided by flaxseed oil	Hypercholesterolemic subjects (Human)	Compared with control, total, LDL & HDL cholesterol levels were reduced by 11, 15.1 & 8.5%. LDL: HDL ratio was reduced by 7·5%.	Gillingham *et al.* (2011)
Diet rich in flaxseed oil was given for 10 days and then a single dose of Cisplatin (6 mg/kg body weight) was administered intraperitoneally while still on diet	Rats	Dietary supplementation of flaxseed oil in Cisplatin (CP)-treated rats ameliorated the CP-induced hepatotoxic and other deleterious effects.	Naqshbandi *et al.* (2012)
Flaxseed powder (60 g/day, 10 g ALA) was administered in a double-blind routine for 12 weeks	Obese population	The total cholesterol level decreased from 197.2 to179.4 mg/dl. LDL&HDL decreased from 122.3 & 50.9 to 106.6 & 47.9 mg/dl, respectively.WhileVLDL increased from 25.8 to 26.6 mg/dl.	Faintuch *et al.* (2011)
Full fatty and partially defatted flaxseed flour @ concentration of 4-20% the supplemented diet was fed for 1 week in the form of unleavened flatbread	Albino rat	12% full fat & 16% defatted flaxseed flour increased TD from 79.4 to 81.45 & 84.6; NPU from 44.3 to 49.4 & 54.65; PER from 1.51 to 1.8& 1.87; and BV from 55.79 to 60.65 & 64.6.	Hussain *et al.* (2012)
30 g/day of flaxseeds were consumed in diet for 3 months	Hypercholesterolemic postmenopausal women	Dietary flaxseed supplementation lowered the total and LDL-cholesterol level, approximately by7% and 10%, respectively. However, the levels of HDL and triglyceride remained unaltered.	Parade *et al.* (2008)
Diet was supplemented daily with 10 g of flaxseed powder for a period of 1 month	Type 2 diabetics	Blood glucose levels were reduced by 19.7%.A favorable reduction in total cholesterol (14.3%), triglycerides (17.5%), LDL-cholesterol(21.8%), and an increase in HDL-cholesterol (11.9%) were also noticed.	Mani *et al.* (2011)
40 g/day of ground flaxseed-containing baked products were fed for 10 weeks	Human	Flaxseed significantly reduced LDL-cholesterol at5 weeks (by 13%), but not at 10 weeks (by 7%)and lipoprotein by a net of 14%. In men, flaxseed reduced HDL-Cholesterol by a net of 16% and9% at 5 and 10 weeks, respectively.	Bloedon *et al.* (2008)

(Table 3) cont.....

Experiment	Model System	Significant Findings	References
One group was fed high cholesterol diet (2 g/100 g) and others were fed the same a diet supplemented with flax/pumpkin seed mixture in the ratio of 5:1	Rats	When compared with the hypercholesterolemic group, flax group showed reduced levels of total cholesterol (220.35 vs 120.48 mg/dL),triacylglycerols (100.93 vs 77.99 mg/dL), VLDL-C (20.19 vs 15.59 mg/dL), LDL-C(171.83 vs 65.37 mg/dL), while increased level of HDL-C from 28.33 to 39.51 mg/dL.	Barakat and Mehmoud (2011)

HERBAL FORMULATION AVAILABLE

Linseed Products

Linseed Oil

Linseed produced in India is utilized mainly for the expression of oil. Bullock-driven ghani and power-driven rotary mills, expellers, and hydraulic presses are used for this purpose. The yield of oil is 28-30% on the weight of seeds. Linseed oil is refined by tanking for a long period. Filtration followed by tanking results in the separation of a part of mucilage. The color of refined oil is improved by treatment with decolorizing agents.

Linseeds Cake/Meal

Linseed cake is obtained as a by-product of the oil. The oil content of the cake varies according to the efficiency of the equipment employed for expelling the oil [45, 53].

Linseed Mucilage

It is prepared from aqueous extract of seeds (soaking in water for 24 hours) precipitation. It is obtained as a white fibrous mass which becomes friable when completely dry.

Linseed Tea

It is also known as an infusion of linseed. Prepared by adding an ounce of the seed in one pint of water, boiled for ten minutes and strained and made preparation with or without the addition of a little liquorice root and sweetened with sugar.

Linseed fibers

Fiber is extracted from the stalks of the plant. Seeds obtained from type grown for fiber are poor in oil content. The color of raw fiber varies from creamy white to grey. Flax-fibers are valued for its outstanding strength, fineness, and durability. It is stronger and more durable than cotton. It is soft, lustrous, and flexible and possesses high water absorbency.

ANTI-NUTRIENTS

Flaxseeds contain anti-nutrients that may have an adverse influence on the health and well-being of the human population. Cyanogenic glycosides are the major anti-nutrients and are fractionated into linustatin (213–352 mg/100 g), neolinustatin (91–203 mg/100 g), linamarin (32 mg/100 g) [46, 47].

DOSAGE

For constipation take 1 tablespoon (10g) of uncrushed or crushed flaxseed 2 - to 3-times daily with plenty of liquid (!). Flax seeds can be taken pre-swelled in water. During therapy with linseed, it must be ensured in each case that there is high fluid intake. To prepare put 5 to 10g of flaxseed in cold water for 20 to 30 min. Thereafter, the liquid is decanted. For external use as a compress, process 30 to 50g of ground flaxseed into a hot and humid pulp [48, 49].

ADVICE

Linseed should not be used if there is a suspicion of intestinal obstruction (ileus) and narrowing of the esophagus and the stomach-intestinal tract as well as in acute inflammatory bowel diseases and disorders of the esophagus and cardia. Use in children under 12 years old **is** not recommended due to a lack of experience [50].

INTERACTION

Linseed should be taken to 1 hour before or after taking other medicines, as otherwise, it may delay the absorption of the other drugs in the gastrointestinal tract [51].

CONCLUSIONS

Based on the information, it is evident that flaxseeds are the richest source of α-linolenic acid and lignans. It is also a considerable potential source of soluble fiber, antioxidants, and high-quality protein. Its long journey from being a medicine in ancient times to health food source in the 21st century has opened the doors for a large population. The role of flaxseed lignans and ω-3 fatty acid in reducing the risks associated with cardiac and coronary disease, cancer (breast, colon, ovary, and prostate), and other human health risk factors have been well known. When a healthy heart is one of the most desired and highly demanded health benefits from functional foods; and where the food industry's goal is to develop innovative solutions to address nutritional challenges, flaxseed is going to play a vital role in the same. Flaxseed can contribute to improving the availability of healthy food choices, specifically by improving the nutrient profile of foods through reductions in the salt, sugar, and saturated fat content; and by increasing the thecontentofω-3 fatty acids and other bioactive compounds. With contribution from such factors, the worldwide market for healthy heart foods is estimated to grow rapidly in the coming years. As a result, flax and flaxseed oil may be preferred ingredients of functional foods and nutraceuticals in the future. There is no doubt that a change to an omega-3 rich and high fiber diet would be beneficial. Therefore the use of flaxseed in whole seed or ground

CONSENT FOR PUBLICATION

Not applicable.

CONFLICT OF INTEREST

The authors confirm that there is no conflict of interest.

ACKNOWLEDGEMENTS

None Declared.

REFERENCES

[1] Murphy PA, Hendrich S. Phytoestrogens in foods. Adv Food Nutr Res 2002; 44: 195-246.
[http://dx.doi.org/10.1016/S1043-4526(02)44005-3] [PMID: 11885137]

[2] ShimYY. Flaxseed (*Linum usitatissimum* L.) compositions and processing: a review. Trends Food Sci Technol 2014; 2(4): 105-10.

[3] Al-Okbi SY. Highlights on functional foods, with special reference to flaxseed. J Nat Fibers 2005; 2(3): 63-8.
[http://dx.doi.org/10.1300/J395v02n03_06]

[4] Carter JF. Potential of flaxseed and flaxseed oil in baked goods and other products in human nutrition. Cereal Foods World 2003; 38(10): 753-9.

[5] Adolphe JL, Whiting SJ, Juurlink BH, Thorpe LU, Alcorn J. Health effects with consumption of the flax lignan secoisolariciresinol diglucoside. Br J Nutr 2010; 103(7): 929-38.
[http://dx.doi.org/10.1017/S0007114509992753] [PMID: 20003621]

[6] Bernacchia R, Preti R, Vinci G. Chemical composition and health benefits of flaxseed. Austin J Nutr Food Sci 2014; 2(8): 1045.

[7] Fedenuik RW, Biliaderis CG. Composition and physiochemical properties of linseed (*Linum usitatissimum*) mucilage. J Agric Food Chem 1994; 42: 240-7.

[http://dx.doi.org/10.1021/jf00038a003]

[8]   Turner TD, Mapiye C, Aalhus JL, *et al.* Flaxseed fed pork: n-3 fatty acid enrichment and contribution to dietary recommendations. Meat Sci 2014; 96(1): 541-7.
[http://dx.doi.org/10.1016/j.meatsci.2013.08.021] [PMID: 24012977]

[9]   AJ Jhala, LM Hall. Flax (*Linum usitatissimum* L.): current uses and future applications. Australian Jof basic and Applied Sci 2010; 4: 4304-12.

[10]   ShimYY. Flaxseed (*Linum usitatissimum* L.) bioactive compounds and peptide nomenclature: A review. Trends Food Sci Technol 2014; 38(1): 5-20.
[http://dx.doi.org/10.1016/j.tifs.2014.03.011]

[11]   Ganorkar PM, Jain RK. Flaxseed—a nutritional punch. Int Food Res J 2013; 20: 519-25.

[12]   Tarpila A, Wennberg T, Tarpila S. Flaxseed as a functional food. Curr Top Nutraceutical Res 2005; 3: 167-88.

[13]   Lunn J, Theobald HE. The health effects of dietary unsaturated fatty acids. British Nutrition Foundation. Nutr Bull 2006; 31: 178-224.
[http://dx.doi.org/10.1111/j.1467-3010.2006.00571.x]

[14]   Rabetafika HN, Remoortel V, Danthine S, *et al.* Flaxseed proteins: food uses and health benefits. Int J Food Sci Technol 2011; 46: 221-8.
[http://dx.doi.org/10.1111/j.1365-2621.2010.02477.x]

[15]   Dev DK, Quensel E. Preparation and functional properties of linseed protein products containing differing levels of mucilage. J Food Sci 1857; 1998(53): 1834-7.

[16]   Alhassane T, Xu XM. Flaxseed lignans: source, biosynthesis, metabolism, antioxidant activity, bio-active components, and health benefits. Compr Rev Food Sci Food Saf 2010; 9: 261-9.
[http://dx.doi.org/10.1111/j.1541-4337.2009.00105.x]

[17]   Malkki Y. Trends in dietary fiber research and development: a review. Acta Aliment 2004; 33: 39-62.
[http://dx.doi.org/10.1556/AAlim.33.2004.1.5]

[18]   Ward WE, Yuan YV, Cheung AM, Thompson LU. Exposure to purified lignan from flaxseed (*Linum usitatissimum*) alters bone development in female rats. Br J Nutr 2001; 86(4): 499-505.
[http://dx.doi.org/10.1079/BJN2001429] [PMID: 11591237]

[19]   Locke CA, Stoll AL. Omega-3 fatty acids in major depression. World Rev Nutr Diet 2001; 89: 173-85.
[http://dx.doi.org/10.1159/000059784] [PMID: 11530734]

[20]   Oomah BD, Mazza G. Flaxseed proteins—a review. Food Chem 1993; 48: 109-14.
[http://dx.doi.org/10.1016/0308-8146(93)90043-F]

[21]   Spiller RC. Pharmacology of dietary fibre. Pharmacol Ther 1994; 62(3): 407-27.
[http://dx.doi.org/10.1016/0163-7258(94)90052-3] [PMID: 7972341]

[22]   Chen J, Saggar JK, Corey P, Thompson LU. Flaxseed cotyledon fraction reduces tumour growth and sensitises tamoxifen treatment of human breast cancer xenograft (MCF-7) in athymic mice. Br J Nutr 2011; 105(3): 339-47.
[http://dx.doi.org/10.1017/S0007114510003557] [PMID: 21138602]

[23]   Mohamed DA, Al-Okbi SY, El-Hariri DM. Mousa. Potential health benefits of bread supplemented with defatted flaxseeds under dietary regimen in normal and type 2 diabetic subjects. Pol J Food Nutr Sci 2012; 62(2): 103-8.
[http://dx.doi.org/10.2478/v10222-011-0049-x]

[24]   Rodriguez-Leyva D, Weighell W, Edel AL, *et al.* Potent antihypertensive action of dietary flaxseed in hypertensive patients. Hypertension 2013; 62(6): 1081-9.
[http://dx.doi.org/10.1161/HYPERTENSIONAHA.113.02094] [PMID: 24126178]

[25]   Tarpila S, Tarpila A, Grohn P, Silvennoinen T, Lindberg L. Efficacy of ground flaxseed on

constipation in patients with irritable bowel syndrome. Curr Top Nutraceutical Res 2004; 2: 119-25.

[26]   Bongoni RN, Sirikonda T, Mekala S, *et al.* Antibacterial and antifungal activities of *Linum usitatissimum* (Flax seeds). Int J Pharm Edu Res 2016; 3(2): 4-8.

[27]   Zanwar AA, Hegde MV, Bodhankar SL. *In vitro* antioxidant activity of ethanolic extract of *Linum usitatissimum*. Pharmacologyonline 2010; 1: 683-96.

[28]   Kaithwas G, Mukherjee A, Chaurasia AK, Majumdar DK. Anti-inflammatory, analgesic and antipyretic activities of *Linum usitatissimum* L. (flaxseed/linseed) fixed oil. Indian J Exp Biol 2011; 49(12): 932-8.
        [PMID: 22403867]

[29]   Dahl WJ, Lockert EA, Cammer AL, Whiting SJ. Effects of flax fiber on laxation and glycemic response in healthy volunteers. J Med Food 2005; 8(4): 508-11.
        [http://dx.doi.org/10.1089/jmf.2005.8.508] [PMID: 16379563]

[30]   Enas FK. Effect of flaxseed application on bone healing in male rats, histological, and immunohisto chemical evaluation of vascular endothelial growth factor. J Med Sci 2017; 17: 81-8.
        [http://dx.doi.org/10.3923/jms.2017.81.88]

[31]   Prasad K. Reduction of serum cholesterol and hypercholesterolemic atherosclerosis in rabbits by secoisolariciresinol diglucoside isolated from flaxseed. Circulation 1999; 99(10): 1355-62.
        [http://dx.doi.org/10.1161/01.CIR.99.10.1355] [PMID: 10077521]

[32]   Prim CR, Baroncini LA, Précoma LB, *et al.* Effects of linseed consumption for a short period of time on lipid profile and atherosclerotic lesions in rabbits fed a hypercholesterolaemic diet. Br J Nutr 2012; 107(5): 660-4.
        [http://dx.doi.org/10.1017/S0007114511003539] [PMID: 21791166]

[33]   Kapoor S, Sachdeva R, Kochhar A. Flaxseed: a potential treatment of lowering blood glucose and lipid profile among diabetic females. Indian J Nutr Diet 2011; 48: 529-36.

[34]   Udenigwe CC, Adebiyi AP, Doyen A, Li H, Bazinet L, Aluko RE. Low molecular weight flaxseed protein-derived arginine-containing peptides reduced blood pressure of spontaneously hypertensive rats faster than amino acid form of arginine and native flaxseed protein. Food Chem 2012; 132(1): 468-75.
        [http://dx.doi.org/10.1016/j.foodchem.2011.11.024] [PMID: 26434317]

[35]   Prasad K. Antihypertensive activity of secoisolariciresinol diglucoside (SDG) isolated from flaxseed: role of guanylatecyclase. Int J Angiol 2004; 13: 7-14.
        [http://dx.doi.org/10.1007/s00547-004-1060-4]

[36]   Marghescu FI, Teodorescu MS, Radu D. The Positive impact of flaxseed (*Linumusitatissimum*) on breast cancer. J Agro Pro Tech 2012; 18(2): 161-8.

[37]   Haidari F, Banaei-Jahromi N, Zakerkish M, Ahmadi K. The effects of flaxseed supplementation on metabolic status in women with polycystic ovary syndrome: a randomized open-labeled controlled clinical trial. Nutr J 2020; 19(1): 8.
        [http://dx.doi.org/10.1186/s12937-020-0524-5] [PMID: 31980022]

[38]   Velasquez MT, Bhathena SJ, Ranich T, *et al.* Dietary flaxseed meal reduces proteinuria and ameliorates nephropathy in an animal model of type II diabetes mellitus. Kidney Int 2003; 64(6): 2100-7.
        [http://dx.doi.org/10.1046/j.1523-1755.2003.00329.x] [PMID: 14633132]

[39]   Bassant MM, Ibrahim AA, *et al.* Study of the protective effect of flaxseed oil on the ethanol-induced gastric mucosal lesion in Non-Overiectomized and ovariectomized Rats. Int J Pharm 2016; 12: 329-39.
        [http://dx.doi.org/10.3923/ijp.2016.329.339]

[40]   Sok DE, Cui HS, Kim MR. Isolation and bioactivities of furfuran type lignan compounds from edible plants. Recent Pat Food Nutr Agric 2009; 1(1): 87-95.
        [http://dx.doi.org/10.2174/2212798410901010087] [PMID: 20653530]

[41]   Fukumitsu S, Aida K, Shimizu H, Toyoda K. Flaxseed lignan lowers blood cholesterol and decreases liver disease risk factors in moderately hypercholesterolemic men. Nutr Res 2010; 30(7): 441-6.
[http://dx.doi.org/10.1016/j.nutres.2010.06.004] [PMID: 20797475]

[42]   Brown L, Caligiuri SPB, Brown D, *et al.* Clinical trials using functional foods provide unique challenges. J Funct Foods 2018; 45: 233-8.
[http://dx.doi.org/10.1016/j.jff.2018.01.024]

[43]   Bassett CM, Rodriguez-Leyva D, Pierce GN. Experimental and clinical research findings on the cardiovascular benefits of consuming flaxseed. Appl Physiol Nutr Metab 2009; 34(5): 965-74.
[http://dx.doi.org/10.1139/H09-087] [PMID: 19935863]

[44]   Mihir P, Thane G, Maddaford J, *et al.* Dietary flaxseed as a strategy for improving human health. Pierce Nutrients 2019; 11(5): 1171.

[45]   Dev DK, Quensel E. Preparation and functional properties of linseed protein products containing differing levels of mucilage. J Food Sci 1988; 53: 1834-7.
[http://dx.doi.org/10.1111/j.1365-2621.1988.tb07854.x]

[46]   Amin T, Thakur M. A comparative study on proximate composition, phytochemical screening, antioxidant and antimicrobial activities of *Linum usitatissimum*L. (flaxseeds). Int J Curr Microbiol Appl Sci 2014; 3: 465-81.

[47]   Dev DK, Quensel E. Functional properties of linseed protein products containing deferent levels of mucilage in selected food systems. J Food Sci 1989; 54: 183-6.
[http://dx.doi.org/10.1111/j.1365-2621.1989.tb08597.x]

[48]   Gambus H, Mikulec A, Gambus F, Pisulewski P. Perspectives of linseed utilization in baking. Pol J Food Nutr Sci 2004; 13(54): 21-7.

[49]   Wang Y, Li D, Wang LJ, Adhikari B. The effect of the addition of flaxseed gum on the emulsion properties of soybean protein isolates (SPI). J Food Eng 2011; 104: 56-62.
[http://dx.doi.org/10.1016/j.jfoodeng.2010.11.027]

[50]   Oomah BD, Mazza G. Processing of flaxseed meal: effect of solvent extraction on physicochemical characteristics. Food Sci Technol (Campinas) 1993; 26: 312-7.

[51]   Hang ZS, Wang LJ, Li D, Li SJ, Ozkan N. Characteristics of flaxseed oil from two different flax plants. Int J Food Prop 2011; 14(6): 1286-96.
[http://dx.doi.org/10.1080/10942911003650296]

[52]   Kajla P, Sharma A, Sood DR. Flaxseed-a potential functional food source. J Food Sci Technol 2015; 52(4): 1857-71.
[http://dx.doi.org/10.1007/s13197-014-1293-y] [PMID: 25829567]

[53]   Goyal A, Sharma V, Upadhyay N, Gill S, Sihag M. Flax and flaxseed oil: an ancient medicine & modern functional food. J Food Sci Technol 2014; 51(9): 1633-53.
[http://dx.doi.org/10.1007/s13197-013-1247-9] [PMID: 25190822]

[54]   Mishra S, Verma P. Flaxseed- Bioactive compounds and health significance. J Humanit Soc Sci 2013; 17(3): 46-50.

SUBJECT INDEX